50 things you can do today to manage back pain

Foreword by Quincy Rabot, osteomyologist and specialist in back pain and sports medicine

Dr Keith Souter

PERSONAL HEALTH GUIDES

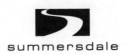

summersdale

50 THINGS YOU CAN DO TODAY TO MANAGE BACK PAIN

Summersdale Publishers Ltd
46 West Street
Chichester
West Sussex
PO19 1RP
UK

www.summersdale.com

Printed and bound in Great Britain

ISBN: 978-1-84953-120-7

Substantial discounts on bulk quantities of Summersdale books are available to corporations, professional associations and other organisations. For details telephone Summersdale Publishers on +44 (0) 1243 771107, fax +44 (0) 1243 786300 or email nicky@summersdale.com.

Disclaimer
Every effort has been made to ensure that the information in this book is accurate and current at the time of publication. The author and the publisher cannot accept responsibility for any misuse or misunderstanding of any information contained herein, or any loss, damage or injury, be it health, financial or otherwise, suffered by any individual or group acting upon or relying on information contained herein. None of the opinions or suggestions in this book are intended to replace medical opinion. If you have concerns about your health, please seek professional advice.

For my good friend Tricia

Acknowledgements

I would like to thank Isabel Atherton, my wonderful agent at Creative Authors who seems to know just when a particular book is needed. Thanks also to Quincy Rabot for kindly agreeing to write a foreword, to Jennifer Barclay, who commissioned this title, and to Chris Turton and Abbie Headon for the helpful editorial input.

It has been a pleasure to work on this book, since the writing process helps to clarify one's clinical knowledge. I hope that it will be useful to anyone with back pain.

Other titles in the Personal Health Guides series include:

50 Things You Can Do Today to Increase Your Fertility
50 Things You Can Do Today to Manage Anxiety
50 Things You Can Do Today to Manage Eczema
50 Things You Can Do Today to Manage Hay Fever
50 Things You Can Do Today to Manage IBS
50 Things You Can Do Today to Manage Insomnia
50 Things You Can Do Today to Manage Migraines
50 Things You Can Do Today to Manage Menopause

Contents

1. Don't panic
2. Learn how the back works
3. Assess the type of back pain that you have
4. Understand the causes of back pain
5. Determine to reduce your risk of back trouble
6. Visit your GP

7. Rest for a short period only
8. Take painkillers
9. Take anti-inflammatories
10. Try a rubefacient
11. Use hot and cold treatment
12. Have a massage

Author's Note

When I was a medical student we were taught a list of causes of back pain. Knowing about them was enough to get through the degree course, yet when one first ventured out into the casualty departments and saw real people with real back pain they were not all that helpful. The surprising thing was that very few of the patients I met were actually affected by any of the causes that we had been taught about. Then, years later in general practice, it was obvious that the undergraduate training about back pain that I had been given was woefully inadequate to deal with the spectrum of back pain that I was seeing, virtually on a daily basis.

About twenty years ago a close relative had a prolapsed intervertebral disc, or as it is commonly (yet incorrectly) known, a slipped disc. He tried all sorts of things to help it before it was finally diagnosed and treated surgically. A talented sportsman, it effectively curtailed his sporting life. Another more distant relative coped with a chronic back condition by doing yoga and regularly visiting a chiropractor. Both of them from time to time asked me for advice and I simply gave them the best advice that I could, although my own understanding of back pain still had a long way to develop.

Then one year I strained my back while bending to pick strawberries. I felt an instant stabbing pain in the small of my back, as if I had been struck from behind by an invisible assailant. I could not move for several minutes and the pain was excruciating. It was as I struggled to get back to normality over the next couple of weeks that I decided to become more knowledgeable about back pain so that I could protect myself against another episode, as well as becoming more effective as a doctor.

I found it to be a difficult task, because people experience back pain in different ways, with differing pain thresholds, different body builds, different occupations and very varied life styles. Yet over the years I built up a range of strategies, looking at first aid measures, lifestyle changes, and different therapies including acupuncture and manipulation. I have found that there is almost always something that you can advise people to do in order to manage their back pain. And I have included the top fifty things in this book for you to start doing today.

Dr Keith Souter

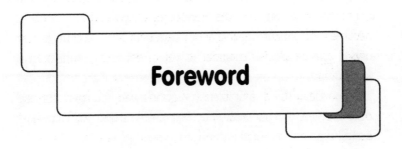

Foreword

**by Quincy Rabot,
Osteomyologist and specialist in
back pain and sports medicine**

If you are reading this the chances are that you suffer from back pain, or have suffered from a bad back in the past.

Next to stress, back pain is the second most common cause of sickness in the UK. Reading this whole book might be one of the best things you can do.

I have noticed that in 30 years of treating back problems the outstanding belief among patients is that the cause of their pain was an event; they lifted something badly, they slipped, they twisted awkwardly or they slept on a bad mattress, and so forth. This is a common misconception. The event was, most likely, only the trigger. The real cause was a complex pattern of musculoskeletal imbalance and dysfunction that had established itself over a period of many years. In such instances, it is only a matter of time before it results in muscle spasm and pain, or worse still, torn ligaments and ruptured or prolapsed discs.

What is most important to understand is that such imbalances in your neuromuscular system can be caused by many aspects of your lifestyle: your mental attitude, your emotional responses to events in your life, your posture and working habits, the sports and exercise you either do or don't do, and even the food you eat.

As I tell my patients, having your episode of back pain treated by a good osteomyologist, chiropractor, osteopath or physiotherapist is like cutting the top off an iceberg. Just because you are out of pain does not mean that the problem has gone away. You need to make some changes to your neuromuscular patterns and work towards regaining good functional patterns to remain pain free.

This calls for some education on how your back works and on what you need to do in order to make the necessary changes. What Dr Keith Souter has done in this clear, splendidly informative and well-thought-out book is to provide you with all the information you need in your journey towards a good, healthy and functional back. All you need to provide is some measure of application and effort!

It is well worth it.

Introduction

Back pain is extremely common. In the UK today more than 2.5 million people regularly experience back pain. Eighty per cent of people will experience at least one episode of back pain at some stage in their life. Surveys published in the *British Medical Journal* in 2000 suggested that in the preceding year up to half of the adult population in the UK had experienced back pain lasting 24 hours. It is the second most common reason for absence from work and currently results in about 9.3 million lost working days per year. No one is immune to it and it can have a dramatic effect on family life, relationships, work and general well-being.

Research from other countries suggests that these figures are not static, but imply that the prevalence of chronic low back pain is steadily rising. A comparison of figures in Colorado, USA, reported in the *Archives of Internal Medicine* in 2009, found that in a 14-year period the prevalence of chronic low back pain rose from 3.9 per cent of adults to 10.2 per cent. Why this should be the case is not clear, yet it is tempting to suppose that it could be related to rising obesity levels in the population, for as we shall see later, this is a significant risk factor.

In terms of cost, the NHS spends over £1 billion a year on back pain treatments. This includes over £500 million on hospital treatment, around £150 million for GP consultations and another £150 million for physiotherapy treatment. In addition to this, it is estimated that over £500 million is also being spent in the private sector for various treatments, both orthodox and complementary.

You would think that with all the money that is being spent we would have all the answers to the problem of back pain. The simple truth, however, is that we do not. Indeed, according to the Royal College of General Practitioners only 15 per cent of cases of back pain are accurately diagnosed.

Please note

This book has been written to help people to manage their back pain. It is not intended as a substitute for medical advice, so readers are advised to check with their GP before undertaking any exercises or taking any of the supplements or remedies mentioned in the text.

Chapter 1

About Back Pain

1. Don't panic

If you do experience an episode of back pain, there is no need to panic. Although it can be painful and may restrict your mobility it is highly likely that it will get better of its own accord in a relatively short time.

While it is natural to worry in case the pain is due to some serious injury or to some underlying condition, in fact most back pain is not serious at all. The vast majority of back pain will improve within two days to two weeks. Most simple back strains do not cause any lasting damage.

It is worth knowing that about half of all the people who experience such an episode of back pain will have another one within two years. The thing is that it can be avoided if you take the correct actions and respect your back.

And helping you to do that is just what this book is about.

2. Learn how the back works

All mammals have the same basic bone structure. Most mammals walk on four legs, but human beings evolved into erect creatures. This was an extremely beneficial adaptation in terms of survival of the species. Speed, balance, manoeuvrability and freeing up of the upper limbs were the result, all useful for a hunter-gatherer creature with the potential to make tools.

The spinal column

The human spinal column seems designed for suppleness and mobility. It is not, however, ideally suited to our sedentary modern lifestyles where we sit in cars or at desks peering at computer screens and so on. We will return to this point later on in the book.

The main functions of the spinal column are weight-bearing and protection of the spinal cord.

Vertebrae

The spinal column is made up of 33 small bones called vertebrae. Five of these are fused to form the sacrum, a triangular structure that forms the back of the pelvis, and four are fused to form the coccyx which continues down from the sacrum as the internal tailbone. Stacked on top of the sacrum are 24 specialised vertebrae, separated from one another by 23 cartilaginous discs. There are seven cervical or neck vertebrae, twelve thoracic or chest vertebrae and five lumbar or lower back vertebrae.

Each vertebra consists of the following parts: a cylindrical body, like a cotton reel or a marshmallow, and an arch that is attached to the body to produce a ring-like structure which encloses the spinal canal.

Each vertebral 'body' provides a strong surface and it is through these and the buffering discs in between that the weight of the body is supported. When you run a finger down someone's spine you will feel the knobbles of their spinous processes.

The different types of vertebrae all have different shapes because they have different roles to play in the spinal column. The lumbar vertebrae are bigger and stronger than the cervical or neck vertebrae, because they have more weight-bearing to do, but they are less mobile.

Intervertebral discs

These are rather like car tyres. They consist of an outer fibrous ring called the annulus fibrosus, which contains a jelly-like pulp called the nucleus pulposus. They are essentially the spinal column's shock absorbers.

Ligaments

The vertebrae are held together by several small fibrous cords called ligaments (from the Latin *ligare*, meaning 'to tie'). In addition, there are two long, very strong ligaments that run the length of the spine, which link the vertebrae and help to hold them in position as a column.

Muscles

The muscles of the back are arranged in three layers:

◗ The superficial or outermost layer consists of trapezius, latissimus dorsi, levator scapulae and the rhomboids. Their purpose is mainly to move the muscles of the upper limbs.

○ The intermediate layer consists of serratus posterior, which has an inferior and a superior part. Their function is mainly to move the ribs to help breathing.

○ The deep layer includes splenius, erector spinae and transversospinales. Their purpose is to move the back.

Curves

A healthy back has three natural curves: a slight forward curve in the neck (cervical curve), a slight backward curve in the upper back (thoracic curve), and a slight forward curve in the low back (lumbar curve). Good posture actually means keeping these three curves in their natural state of balanced alignment.

Spinal cord and spinal nerves

The spinal cord and the brain make up the central nervous system. The spinal cord extends down through the spinal canal formed by the vertebrae for a distance of about eighteen inches. It then extends downwards as the cauda equina, so called because it resembles a horse's tail.

Spinal nerves emerge from the cord through special canals to supply the various parts of the body. Thus:

○ Cervical nerves supply the head and neck.

○ A mix of cervical and thoracic nerves supply the upper limbs.

○ Thoracic nerves supply the chest and abdomen.

○ Lumbar nerves supply the trunk and the legs.

○ Sacral and coccygeal nerves supply the pelvic area.

When any of these nerves are affected they can produce back pain in the area of the back that they supply. Thus pressure on cervical nerve roots will cause neck pain, pressure on lumbar nerve roots will give low back pain, and sacral nerve root pressure can give pain in the buttocks.

3. Assess the type of back pain that you have

It is important, initially, to differentiate acute from chronic pain. Many people mistakenly think that 'acute' and 'chronic' are two poles of a spectrum of experience. This is not the case. They are two entirely different types of pain.

Acute pain
This is the expected physiological response to a stimulation which the body perceives to be unpleasant. The simplest example is the immediate reflex withdrawal of your hand when you burn your fingers. If the burn is mild, the pain will go on for a relatively short period of time. This type of pain is seen to have a useful purpose, in that it alerts the body to a problem that it can readily relieve. It causes the individual to take action to avoid further injury or damage.

'Recurrent pain' describes repeated episodes of pain. This is the type that you get with repeated attacks of back pain.

Chronic pain
This is the continual experience of an unpleasant sensation which is unlikely to disappear of its own accord. This is the typical background pain of, say, arthritis. Unlike acute pain, this type of pain has no

useful biological function. It just grinds away at you and can, if you allow it, seriously impair your quality of life.

If back pain lasts for more than 12 weeks it is considered to be chronic back pain.

The point is that these two types of pain (acute and chronic) may actually have different mechanisms and different pathways to the brain, where they are perceived as 'pain.' Acute pain is going to get better in time, albeit that it may come again as a recurrent pain. Chronic pain, on the other hand, is by definition on-going, and the individual is going to need to develop strategies to cope with it. This may include medication, but it is unlikely that this will be the whole answer.

It is a somewhat arbitrary differentiation, but back pain is sometimes categorised according to the duration of the pain.

Pain categories

Acute back pain – less than 6 weeks
Sub-acute back pain – 6 to 12 weeks
Chronic back pain – 12 weeks or more

---

4. Understand the causes of back pain

Most back pains are experienced in the low back or lumbar area. This is because it is the power base of the back, which is heavily muscled and through which weight-bearing occurs for walking, standing, bending and lifting. The neck is the next most common part of the spine to be affected by pain. The thoracic spine is not an area that is often strained, although it can be subject to problems as a result of degenerative changes caused by osteoarthritis.

Some common causes of back pain

Sprains and strains

These are the most common causes of low back pain. One can usually pinpoint the cause as the result of a lifting injury, a problem during bending, a sneeze or cough that provoked a sudden episode of pain, or some other kind of sudden physical exertion.

The old name 'lumbago' is still used for low back pain that does not radiate beyond the low back. It is a non-specific diagnosis. The problem comes from strain on muscles or ligaments in the back, although it is almost impossible to differentiate the two on clinical examination. It may produce severe pain, but the severity of pain does not in itself mean that it is serious. It usually ends within a period ranging from two days to six weeks.

Myofascial pain

This is pain occurring in the muscles, arising from 'trigger points' within particular muscles. These are small hyper-sensitive areas within the muscles, which often coincide with the development of little nodules. Myofascial pain is often characterised by pain radiating from the trigger point. It can mimic other conditions and is a common cause of pseudo-sciatica; that is, it produces back pain and radiation of pain down the leg, but without any alteration in reflexes.

It is a common cause of chronic back pain and is usually amenable to massage, physiotherapy and acupuncture.

Fibromyalgia syndrome
This is a complex condition where the individual can experience muscular pain anywhere in the body, including the back. The muscles may be quite tender and movement may be limited. It usually builds up and worsens over a few weeks. Most medical investigations will prove negative, but it is important to establish the diagnosis, for it can be the underlying cause of a chronic back problem.

Disc problems
Although people often fear that they may have 'slipped a disc', in actual fact discs do not slip. What can happen is that a disc can bulge, rather in the same way that a car tyre can bulge if there is a weakness in the wall. In this case there may be some irritation on surrounding tissues or nerve roots.

Sometimes a disc can 'prolapse', meaning that the annulus fibrosus, the fibrous ring that resembles the car tyre, partially ruptures to allow some of the inner jelly-like nucleus pulposus to seep out. If this happens near a nerve it will irritate it and pain will be felt down the course of the nerve.

Both of these cases can cause sciatica, by irritating the sciatic nerve, which is the main nerve supplying the leg. Sciatica is the name for a condition in which the sciatic nerve is compressed or irritated by inflammation, the result being pain travelling down the leg. It is a complex nerve formed from several lumbar and sacral nerve roots. The actual distribution of the pins and needles sensation or pain that is felt can guide a doctor to diagnose which disc is pressing on which nerve root or roots.

Joint degeneration
Arthritis in the spinal column can result in bony outgrowths forming on vertebrae, erosion of cartilage and drying and shrinking of discs. In addition, the small facet joints which allow the vertebrae to glide

and move may be affected. This is usually a result of osteoarthritis, which is generally considered to be a type of wear-and-tear problem of all joints.

Facet syndrome is a situation where one or more of the facet joints become inflamed, causing the back to lock up. It can occur very suddenly when bending, almost as if one has been kicked in the small of the back by some unseen individual.

Osteoporosis

In older people, the condition 'osteoporosis' or 'thinning of the bones' can produce pain in the thoracic spine, effectively the upper back. Everyone tends to lose calcium from their bones as they get older, but in some people this loss is excessive. Women after the menopause are especially prone to this, so it is a good idea to have this checked by your doctor if you think you are at risk.

The loss of bone mass can predispose people to fractures of the wrist, hips and thoracic vertebrae. The thoracic vertebrae can become distorted or compressed at one edge, rather like a marshmallow, and effectively collapse. This happens in 'crush fractures' of the thoracic spine and results in very sudden, severe pain. As a result of the worsening osteoporosis there may be a tendency for the sufferer to stoop forward, eventually producing the so-called 'dowager's hump' of old age.

Risk factors for osteoporosis

- **Family history** – if one of your parents had a hip fracture you may be at risk.

- **Age** – bone loss increases with age. Over the age of 75 years, 50 per cent of the population have osteoporosis.

◯ **Sex** – females are more prone to develop osteoporosis.

◯ **Smoking** – this is one of the greatest risk factors.

◯ **Low body weight** – a low BMI of 19 or less is a significant risk for osteoporosis.

◯ **Past history of fractures** – if you have easily broken bones in the past then you may be at risk.

◯ **Hormone problems** – the female hormone oestrogen protects bones, but when the level drops at the menopause the protection goes. Early menopause is therefore a risk, as is a history of hysterectomy where the ovaries have been removed. So too is a history of overactive thyroid and parathyroid glands.

◯ **Malabsorption conditions** – these are conditions that may be associated with diminished absorption of calcium from the food. For example, coeliac disease or Crohn's disease.

◯ **Other conditions** – rheumatoid arthritis, diabetes, HIV, chronic respiratory disease or a history of organ transplantation.

◯ **Drugs** – some prescribed medication can predispose towards osteoporosis, including: long term steroids by mouth (longer than three months), anti-epileptic drugs, breast cancer drugs, prostate cancer drugs.

Other diseases

As mentioned above, osteoarthritis is the most common type of arthritis and is considered to be a wear and tear problem. There are other types of arthritis, such as rheumatoid arthritis, where the problem is inflammation. This is characterised by early morning stiffness, which improves slightly as one gets moving. Back pain is not usually the earliest symptom, but it may need to be excluded, as should other related conditions.

Polymyalgia rheumatica is an inflammatory condition of the muscles, mainly affecting the shoulder and pelvic girdles. It classically presents itself in middle age, literally overnight, so that the individual cannot get up in the morning or cannot raise their arms to do their hair. With such a dramatic onset, an early medical opinion is advised.

Not all back pain arises from the spine or from the causes mentioned above. Kidney infections, bowel disorders and even malignant conditions of organs such as the thyroid, kidney, breast, prostate and ovary can all spread to bone. While these account for only a small percentage of back pains, they do need to be diagnosed early, so one should take note of 'red light' warning symptoms, which we shall look at shortly (See item 6. Visit your GP)

5. Determine to reduce your risk of back trouble

The following factors increase the risk of back pain:

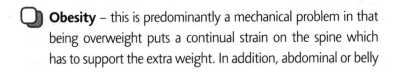 **Smoking** – this is the greatest risk to health in general. Smoking reduces the body's ability to repair itself; it actually promotes inflammation and it interferes with the absorption of calcium.

Obesity – this is predominantly a mechanical problem in that being overweight puts a continual strain on the spine which has to support the extra weight. In addition, abdominal or belly fat will tend to pull the body forward, thereby throwing extra strain on the spine.

Congenital structural problems – some people are born with defects in the structure of the individual vertebrae, the pelvis or the limbs. Anything which causes the body to adopt a posture that is not symmetrical will predispose to back pain.

Scoliosis – this is a sidewards bend in the back. It will inevitably cause the body to bear weight in an uneven manner.

Older age – there is increased bone loss with age, effectively thinning the bones.

Being female – the bones in females are generally smaller and thinner.

Strenuous work – this is liable to cause wear and tear on the skeleton.

Being sedentary – this causes weakness of the supporting muscles.

Stressful occupation – with increased stress the body is less able to repair itself and inflammatory processes are more likely.

Anxiety – it is well recognised by GPs that anxious people are more likely to experience painful conditions.

Depression – similar to anxiety, depression seems to lower the threshold for pain, so that painful conditions including back pain are more common.

Of the above factors there are only two (the inherited medical conditions and age) you cannot readily change with a concentrated effort. If you think that you have any of these risk factors then you should strive to reduce them, or seek help in order to do so.

6. Visit your GP

Most back pain gets better in a few weeks, whether you see a doctor or not. If the pain is severe and is not getting better after a few days, despite painkillers, then it is reasonable to seek a medical opinion from your GP. Certainly, if it has not improved after four weeks it is time to go. And of course, if the pain started with a fall and you think that you could have fractured something then you should go straight to a casualty department.

Your doctor will try to diagnose your back pain on the basis of the history of your complaint and a physical examination. This will involve looking at and assessing the area of pain, its severity, and how it is affecting you physically. Your back will be examined for tenderness and any alteration in sensation, power, mobility or your reflexes.

If necessary, blood tests will be arranged to exclude any inflammatory arthritic condition, or any other disorder.

The following tests may also be arranged:

Plain X-ray of the back – looking for any evidence of arthritis. This is one of the simplest tests, but it is of limited value since most back pain causes will not show up.

○ **CT scan** – this stands for computerised tomography. It is essentially a computerised method of assessing a series of X-rays taken from different angles in order to try and build up a series of visual slices of your back. Again, it is of limited value in the diagnosis of a back pain, but is of more value in eliciting evidence of underlying disease.

○ **DEXA scan** – this is a bone densitometry scan, done on the lower spine and the hips and sometimes the wrists as well, in order to determine the density of the bones. This is important to determine the presence or the risk of developing osteoporosis.

○ **MRI scan** – this stands for magnetic resonance imaging. This is an incredibly sophisticated investigation which uses magnetism, ultrasound and computerised technology to build up multiple images of the inside of the body. This may show changes in joints that do not show up on X-rays, and can be a useful diagnostic tool in the early stages of rheumatoid arthritis. It also shows up soft tissues. It can be an alarming investigation for people who are prone to claustrophobia, since with some scanners it involves passing through a large, tunnel-like apparatus.

As mentioned earlier, a specific diagnosis is only likely to be made in about 15 per cent of cases of back pain. The main thing is to exclude underlying problems and to spot any cause that may require further referral to a specialist, or other health professional, such as a physiotherapist or osteopath.

Very few people with back pain will require surgery. Nine out of ten people with a prolapsed disc will find that their symptoms settle within six weeks. One in ten may need surgery and an assessment by a surgeon would be sensible at that time.

Red light warning symptoms

If any of the following symptoms are present a medical opinion should be sought as a matter of urgency.

- If you have a history of cancer – there is always the possibility of a secondary tumour or multiple tumours from the cancer spreading to bone.

- If you are suddenly incontinent – this demands urgent treatment, because it can indicate that a disc has prolapsed internally to affect the spinal cord within the spinal canal.

- The development of numbness, tingling or pins and needles down one or both legs. These would indicate that there is nerve root irritation and it merits investigation by your GP.

- Any urinary symptoms, such as an increase in the need to pass urine. There is the possibility that a urinary infection or a urinary calculus (stone) could be causing the back pain. This is especially the case if a high temperature is present.

Your GP might prescribe painkillers and anti-inflammatory drugs, and issue a sick note if necessary.

It is worth discussing a management plan together, so that you know just when to return if necessary. Such a plan includes the likely course of the condition, the things that you should and should not do, the time scale for returning to exercise and the reason for particular types of medication and the method of taking them. This is all very important, since the aim is to ensure that an acute back problem does not develop into a chronic one. Above all, you need to be an active participant in this management plan, not merely the recipient of drugs.

Chapter 2

First Aid for
Acute Back Pain

There are several first aid measures that you can begin at the start of an episode of back pain. If you do the right things then you will probably ease the pain and reduce the length of the episode.

7. Rest for a short period only

When I entered general practice in 1978 the standard advice for back pain was bed rest, sometimes for a week and sometimes for months on end. The theory was that you rested the weight-bearing spinal column, thereby allowing inflammation to settle down and pain to go.

This is utterly refuted these days, except for a day or two at most at the start of an episode of back pain. The evidence is that prolonged bed rest is bad for you and can cause the following:

Stiffness

You know that even when your back is well, the first thing you have to do on getting up in the morning is have a good stretch. This eases normal stiffness. Prolonged bed rest worsens this effect.

Muscle weakness

This is very apparent even after a week. Muscle strength lessens and the muscles will start to become smaller – so-called 'muscle wasting'.

Bone weakness

Calcium is lost from bones and prolonged bed rest can increase the risk of osteoporosis.

Fitness drops

This is an inevitable result of the muscles weakness. But also, because you are not stretching your cardiovascular system your overall fitness drops.

Anxiety

We are now well aware that prolonged bed rest actually makes people feel anxious. They will feel anxious about important things that are not getting done, worry that they are not contributing to the family, and perhaps start to fear that their job could be at risk. Also, it is common to become anxious that recovery is not going to take place. This increase in anxiety can actually make pain worse and can delay recovery.

Depression

It is common to feel bored and down in the dumps when forced to stay in bed for more than a couple of days. If one is also experiencing problems with a back pain that doesn't seem to get better with bed rest then this can turn into clinical depression. As with anxiety, depression can make pain harder to deal with. It also becomes hard to fend off the apathy that comes with depression.

Thrombosis

This is a serious risk from prolonged bed rest. A blood clot can form in the deep veins of the calf muscles. This is called DVT or deep vein thrombosis. If this develops there is a very real risk that part of the clot could break off and be pumped to the lungs to cause a pulmonary embolism. This is potentially fatal.

Ulceration

Prolonged immobility can cause skin ulceration on pressure points such as the heels and the small of the back.

So, no more than two days in bed! And when you do lie it is better to lie on your side or on your back with your knees bent and resting on a pillow or cushion.

8. Take painkillers

Acute pain needs relief. People often think that painkillers merely mask the pain, so they worry that they could injure themselves further by doing something while they are unable to feel pain. In fact, you will not do any further damage: your body will not permit you to. The muscles would tend to go into complete spasm and stop you from moving if you happened to exert them.

During an acute episode of pain it is quite all right to take a simple painkiller, such as paracetamol, which you can buy over the counter. It is best to avoid aspirin, since it is a gastric irritant.

Take one or two paracetamol at a time every 4 to 6 hours, or follow the dosage instructions on the box. It is better to get the pain under control in an acute episode of back pain rather than waiting until it is unbearable. Note that I am referring to acute episodes here. Chronic back pain control is a different matter and I shall come to that in the next chapter.

It is probable that you will not need to take the painkillers for any more than three or four days.

TENS

Another possible aid to relieve back pain is a Transcutaneous Electrical Nerve Stimulation (TENS) machine. This is something to consider if your doctor feels it would help.

A TENS unit is about the size of a personal stereo. It is battery charged and delivers a small electrical current via wires to sticky pad electrodes that are placed over the area of pain. The electrodes and wires can be worn under normal clothing and the TENS unit may be clipped onto clothing or carried in a pocket.

There are two mechanisms by which this system is thought to reduce pain: firstly, when it is used at high frequency to stimulate certain non-pain-transmitting nerves, it effectively overrides the pain signals from the pain-sensing nerves; and secondly, when used at low frequencies it is thought to cause the release of endorphins, which are the body's natural painkilling chemicals.

The device is used for about 15 minutes at a time, several times a day, rather than continuously.

It should not be used by anyone who has not had their pain diagnosed, nor should it be used by anyone suffering from epilepsy, or anyone with a pacemaker fitted. Also, it should not be used without supervision by anyone who is pregnant, though it is sometimes used during labour as a method of pain relief.

9. Take anti-inflammatories

An anti-inflammatory drug like ibuprofen may help. It can either be taken on its own, or with a simple painkiller like paracetamol. It is best not to take any of the combination painkillers (tablets or capsules containing combinations of drugs like aspirin, codeine or caffeine) at the same time as anti-inflammatories without checking with your own doctor.

Ibuprofen belongs to a group of drugs called the non-steroidal anti-inflammatory drugs, or NSAIDs. This means that they have a similar anti-inflammatory effect to steroids, yet they do not have many of the side effects of steroids.

The dose for ibuprofen is 200 to 400 mg three times a day. As with painkillers you probably will not need to take them for more than a few days.

They should be avoided in the following circumstances:

If you have a history of stomach problems, like indigestion or an ulcer. They have a potential gastric irritant effect and can in a small number of people cause bleeding into the stomach.

If you are taking aspirin. Both ibuprofen and aspirin have gastric irritant potential so there would be a real risk of producing bleeding into the stomach by taking both at the same time.

If you are taking anti-coagulant (blood thinning) drugs, because of the risk of haemorrhage.

If you are pregnant. The effects of any drug on the developing baby are uncertain and all drugs should be avoided, except on the advice of your doctor or midwife.

If you are asthmatic. The NSAID group of drugs can all provoke an episode of asthma.

10. Try a rubefacient

Most chemists have a section selling various preparations which can be rubbed on, and which are promoted for the easing of sprained muscles and to treat acute lumbago and non-specific back pain. There is a bewildering array of them, revelling in names evocative of the medicine of yesteryear. You will find gels, creams, embrocations, liniments and balms. The National Institute for Clinical Excellence (NICE), a body which advises doctors on the evidence for various treatments, concluded that there was little hard evidence of the efficacy of such preparations for acute injuries and back pains. It suggested that their value was simply that they contained a rubefacient.

A rubefacient is an agent that produces heat. It is derived from the Latin word *rubor*, meaning heat. This seems to be the reaction that many of these rubbing-on preparations induce; they produce local heat or irritation of the skin over the area, which then overrides pain signals from the deeper tissues. This is actually a quite legitimate mechanism of pain relief called 'counter-irritation'.

OVDO – Olympic Victor's Dark Ointment

Interestingly, an ancient medical treatise from the first century AD has recently been unearthed by the British Museum. It details how to make a remedy which in Latin was called *'Fuscum olympionico inscriptum'*. This translates as 'Olympic Victor's Dark Ointment'. This was purportedly a liquid plaster which had cooling and painkilling effects, and which reduced inflammation and bruising.

This is a fascinating find, since it shows that sports medicine was alive and well in the ancient world. And an effective painkilling, anti-inflammatory remedy would have been worth its weight in gold to treat injuries in the gladiatorial circus or in the athletics arena.

This particular treatise was written by the Greek physician Claudius Galenus of Pergamum (AD 131 to 201), who is known to history as Galen. He worked in a gladiator school, later becoming physician to the emperor Marcus Aurelius. He was the first anatomist and the most influential medical writer for a thousand years.

He wrote about OVDO and recommended it as being of great benefit for bruises and black eyes.

Researchers from the British Museum and the University of Copenhagen have reproduced the remedy and tested its efficacy. It consisted of the following ingredients: antimony, cadmia, saffron, frankincense, myrrh, acacia, gummi, opium, pompholyx, aloe indica and raw egg. The various ingredients would help to soothe inflammation and pain, reduce swelling and promote healing, with the egg acting as a binding agent.

The research team found that when they made it up it would have been too gritty to apply to the eye, but that it could have been applied to the face and other parts of the body. It was a semi-liquid which set like a modern spray-on flexible plaster. Amazingly, it was about 25 per cent as effective as a modern pain-relieving patch. They also found that it delivered pain relief quite rapidly, but also had a slow-release effect, rather like present slow-relief plasters. The antimony was a concern, since repeated use of it could result in toxic levels accumulating in the body, but used short-term, it would have a cooling and anti-inflammatory effect.

I mention this here to illustrate that pain relief and anti-inflammation have been prime concerns of doctors across the centuries, and that even in antiquity they had medicines that were effective.

Opodeldoc

Not long after I started work in General Practice I found myself struggling to help a patient with back pain. I had tried several types of painkiller and anti-inflammatory drugs, but without any success in controlling his problem. One day he strode into the consulting room, bent and touched his toes, then slapped an old bottle on the desk.

'Deldoc,' he said. 'That's what you need to give folk to rub on their backs. It cured me.'

To cut a long story short, it was an evil-smelling embrocation that a farmer friend of his had given him. I did not recognise the name, but I subsequently found out that it was actually called 'opodeldoc.' To my surprise I learned that it was a camphorated soap liniment, usually fortified with various herbs and oils, which had been devised by a physician known as Paracelsus in the sixteenth century. His actual name was Theophrastus Bombastus von Hohenheim, but he had chosen the name Paracelsus, which meant 'greater than Celsus'.

This patient and his opodeldoc convinced me that rubbing on agents could indeed be useful.

Embrocations, liniments, gels and balms

You will find many preparations, such as Deep Heat, Tiger Balm and Dog Oil available over the counter at chemists and health shops. These are all rubefacients and are variants on the OVDO of Roman times and the opodeldoc of the sixteenth century. They are all used to apply to the skin. Lotions are liquids, which are simply applied to the skin surface and left. A liniment or embrocation is also a liquid, but it is applied with a degree of friction, so it is rubbed into the skin. Gels and balms tend to be more viscous, and are like creams and ointments. They too are usually rubbed in.

Most liniments contain alcohol or acetone, or some other solvent which quickly evaporates when it touches the skin. This produces a slight cooling and soothing effect. They also contain one or more irritant substances which will produce an irritation in the skin and which may stimulate the blood vessels in the tissues to dilate. This causes a counter-irritation effect. This means that by producing an irritation in the local tissues, the nervous system over-rides the pain signals that are coming from the deeper tissues. The rubbing also has this effect, so it also contributes to this counter-irritation to reduce the pain.

Non-steroidal rubefacients

Some creams and gels contain non-steroidal agents, such as ibuprofen. In addition to the normal counter-irritant mode of action these also deliver a small amount of anti-inflammatory drug which can be absorbed through the skin.

People with asthma or people who are taking anticoagulants should avoid using these preparations, because there is a risk that they could cause a worsening of asthma or cause bleeding. Pregnant women should also avoid them because there is always that risk that any drug could affect the developing baby inside her.

Capsaicin

Some rubefacients contain capsaicin, which is the active ingredient from cayenne or red chilli peppers. It is definitely known to have anti-inflammatory effects and is an extremely potent rubefacient. It is available on prescription from your doctor and comes in two strengths. It should be taken as your doctor suggests. It should be avoided if you are allergic to chillies.

Arnica

This is a remedy often used for bruises and traumas in homoeopathic medicine. Arnica gel or cream is also available over the counter. In my experience this works extremely well and is soothing when applied to the back during an acute episode.

How often can rubefacients be used?

Generally, rubefacients can be applied two to four times a day.

11. Use hot and cold treatment

You will find immense variation in opinion among health practitioners about the merits or otherwise of hot and cold treatment. My own view is that both heat and cold treatments are valuable, but that their benefits vary from person to person. This is perfectly understandable, since we are all individuals with unique ways of reacting.

We can, however, make a few general points.

Be safe

This is of paramount importance. Always be sure that you are applying the treatments safely, and be particularly careful about applying packs or water bottles directly to the skin. The skin can be damaged by both heat and cold. It is always sensible to use a towel between a heat pack or a cold pack and the skin.

The basic principle

Cold is good for reducing inflammation. Heat is useful for easing pain and stiffness.

Cold treatments

◯ Cold will tend to cause blood vessels to constrict, which is the desired effect when treating inflamed tissue.

◯ The logical thing to do after an acute injury, like a twist or a wrench of the back, is to use cold to reduce inflammation. The cold also will produce numbness, so it will have a pain-relieving effect as well.

◯ Use cold repeatedly in the first 24 to 48 hours after an acute injury.

◯ You can use a pack of frozen peas wrapped in a towel, or crush ice in a plastic bag, or fill a hot water bottle with ice or iced water.

◯ Take care about using ice for too long. As a rule of thumb, five to ten minutes is the ideal time to apply cold and 20 minutes is the longest you should ever apply cold continuously.

◯ Always inspect the skin and make sure it does not get excessively white. If the back starts to hurt more, then remove the cold pack.

Heat treatments

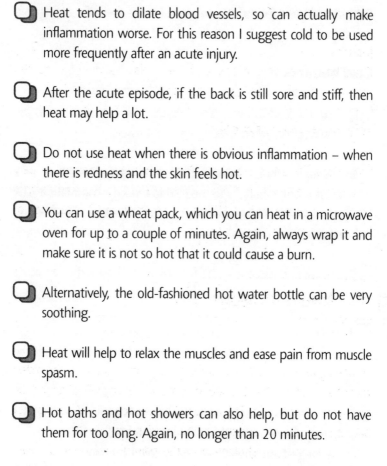

Heat tends to dilate blood vessels, so can actually make inflammation worse. For this reason I suggest cold to be used more frequently after an acute injury.

After the acute episode, if the back is still sore and stiff, then heat may help a lot.

Do not use heat when there is obvious inflammation – when there is redness and the skin feels hot.

You can use a wheat pack, which you can heat in a microwave oven for up to a couple of minutes. Again, always wrap it and make sure it is not so hot that it could cause a burn.

Alternatively, the old-fashioned hot water bottle can be very soothing.

Heat will help to relax the muscles and ease pain from muscle spasm.

Hot baths and hot showers can also help, but do not have them for too long. Again, no longer than 20 minutes.

Saunas

A sauna is an excellent type of treatment for stiffness. The dry heat of the sauna usually loosens up stiff muscles and joints. If you have high blood pressure or a heart problem, you should always check with your doctor before using a sauna.

Turkish bath

A Turkish bath supplies moist heat and also seems to be beneficial to many people with back pain.

Jacuzzi

If you have access to one, this can be very relaxing when the muscles are sore and stiff. Do not stay longer than 20 minutes.

Alternating hot and cold

Some people find that alternating hot and cold works more effectively than either alone. I think that this makes sense and I generally advise five-minute sessions of each, alternating them in the sequence of hot, to cold, to hot, to cold, to hot.

12. Have a massage

A massage is a natural treatment for back pain. It is one of the oldest forms of treatment in the world, since to rub a hurt is almost an instinctive thing to do. The ancient Chinese advocated massage for back pain, as did the ancient Greek physician Hippocrates.

Gentle rubbing or stroking over the painful area, with a cream like arnica, or just some simple olive oil can be done by any willing volunteer. If it is no more than this then no harm can be done.

The action of rubbing stimulates the circulation of the lymph system, which runs parallel with the circulatory system, so it encourages removal of debris and products of inflammation by the lymphatic system.

A more professional massage from a remedial therapist or physiotherapist can be very helpful and may speed up recovery during an acute back pain episode.

We will return to massage in the very last tip in the book, when we are considering the management of recurrent or chronic back pain.

Chapter 3

Pain Management

Pain is an enigma. It is not an entity in itself, but an unpleasant experience. When a pain has gone, you cannot reproduce it just by thinking about it. You can recollect that it was unpleasant and that it made you feel a particular way. You can even describe what it felt like, but you cannot consciously bring it back to mind so that you can experience it.

In Chapter 1 we looked at the way that we classify the different types of pain. That is helpful in terms of trying to work out how best to deal with it. Acute pain is far easier to deal with than chronic pain, as most people with a chronic or recurrent back problem will be well aware. The truth is that pain is one of the greatest challenges faced in medical practice, and in the instance of chronic back pain it may help to adopt some alternative strategies.

13. Understand how pain is perceived

It is helpful to try to picture the way that your brain perceives pain. It is your brain that perceives where all the parts of your body are at any one time, and if a particular part is producing a pain signal the brain perceives this and you 'feel' the pain in that part.

Pain pathways

The actual route by which a pain stimulus is transmitted to the brain in acute pain is quite well established.

All over and throughout the body there are tiny sensors called nociceptors. The word is derived from the Latin *nocere*, meaning 'to injure'. They were first described in 1906, by Sir Charles Scott Sherrington, professor of physiology at Oxford University. It was an extremely important discovery, for which he received a Nobel Prize. These nociceptors react to all injurious or harmful stimuli and they are the first step in the process. In back pain a great number of these nociceptors may be stimulated in joints, muscles and tendons.

The nociceptor then sends an impulse up a nerve along a particular pain pathway. One of the main pathways is called the spino-thalamic tract. The impulse that is sent up a nerve from the nociceptor reaches a neuron (nerve cell) in the dorsal horn of the spinal cord, which is at the back of the cord. This nerve cell transmits the impulse across to the opposite side of the spinal cord where it joins with another nerve cell, which then sends the impulse up the cord to a part of the brain called the thalamus, at the base of the brain. From there, other nerve cells transmit the impulse up to higher parts of the brain where it is interpreted as a pain.

The spino-thalamic tract is responsible for transmitting pain, temperature sensation and fine touch sensation, which explains why pains may be experienced as hot or cold. Similarly, the pins and needles sensation that accompanies some pains is accountable by combined stimulation of the fine touch and pain nerve fibres.

Once pain is perceived, appropriate action can be taken by the individual to allay the painful stimulus. One can see how this can operate in acute pain, such as when one's finger is burned on a hot object. The brain tells the body to take evasive action. But chronic pain is different and altogether more complex.

Brain studies

We are fortunate today in having two very effective types of scanners, called functional Magnetic Resonance Imaging (fMRI) and Positive Emission Tomography (PET), which allow researchers to build a picture of what is happening inside the brain during certain activities or when someone is thinking different types of thought.

Work at the North-Western University's Feinberg School of Medicine in Chicago has recently helped to unravel some of the mystery of chronic pain using fMRI scans. The research team were actually able to demonstrate that acute and chronic pain light up different parts of the brain.

In acute pain, such as occurs with a burned finger, or an acute muscle strain, there is intense activity within the thalamus, a sort of switchboard within the brain. By contrast, chronic back pain lights up the prefrontal cortex at the front of the brain and the limbic system in the middle of the brain. The prefrontal cortex is involved in higher thought processing, and the limbic system is part of the brain that seems to be involved in emotions.

They also found that the longer a person has been experiencing chronic pain the more activity occurs in the prefrontal cortex. This rather implies that the brain then holds a memory of the pain that can be replayed again and again. It also implies that the emotional aspect of the pain will tend to be replayed at the same time.

The significance of this is that drugs are not necessarily going to solve the problem of a chronic pain condition. They may suppress parts of the perception of the pain, yet they will do nothing for that part which is laid down as a memory trace, or which has an emotional memory. This very much fits in with the experience of people who have developed a chronic back problem.

The human pain matrix

A current concept in medicine which has been developed from the work of Ronald Melzack and Patrick Wall is the human pain matrix, a widespread neurological network that is involved in the perception of all types of pain. It seems to have two main components which operate in parallel with each other. The inner one is called the 'medial pain system' which processes the emotional side of pain, that is, anxiety, fear and stress. The outer one is called the 'lateral pain system' and it is responsible for processing the physical sensations, such as the intensity of the pain, its localisation in the body and its duration.

Another piece of research from the University of Manchester used PET to investigate how the brain processes the experience of pain in arthritis. The researchers looked at arthritic pain because it tends to produce morning stiffness and joint aches, and is subject to flare-ups. In other words, arthritic pains tend to be acute and intermittent, as well as having the background chronic pain. For this reason, it is possible to compare arthritic pain with artificial or experimental pain (pain deliberately induced in an experiment by pressure or heat).

In this study, patients with osteoarthritis, the most common type of arthritis, were examined in order to see what happened in their brains during episodes of arthritic pain and episodes of artificial experimental pain. They all had PET scans performed during three types of pain condition: during arthritic knee pain; during artificial pain from the application of heat; and when they were pain-free.

It was found that the pain matrix was inactive when they were free of pain, but it was activated when pain was experienced, whether it was acute or chronic. During arthritic pain, however, the medial pain system was predominantly activated. This suggests that during a flare-up there is a significant emotional accompaniment to the pain. The individual's brain seems to reflect fear, stress and distress, in varying degrees. In contrast, artificial pain predominantly affects the lateral pain system, or mainly produces a physical response. Artificial pain has no emotional component, presumably because the person knows that it is artificial and that it will go away.

This shows that even though someone may know that an acute flare-up of arthritis will probably go away eventually, they worry that it might continue, or even get worse, and so the pain induces those thoughts and emotions.

This emotional component of pain is potentially very important because it suggests that the role of the mind in pain control can be crucial.

14. Use your imagination as a painkiller

In 2002 I attended a very interesting photographic exhibition at St Thomas's Hospital in London. The theme was chronic pain. I thought it was an extremely clever idea because it introduced an artistic perspective to the enigma of pain.

The photographs in the exhibition were portrayals of people's perceptions of their pain. One photograph showed a concrete straitjacket that the artist had made to illustrate one person's experience and perception. To this person pain was a solid thing, a constricting and isolating thing. And it weighed him down, just as concrete would.

Other images showed red-hot wires glowing in the dark, animal scratches on stone, and gloves full of crawling ants. You can imagine the quality of the pain those people were experiencing; the various artworks showed that no two people experience the same pain. It has a unique feel and, if you think about the concept of the pain matrix, there is a unique blend of emotions associated with it.

The imagery that can be used to describe a pain, therefore, gives you a means of using your imagination as a painkiller. When you have a pain, try to imagine what your pain looks like in a symbolic manner like this. Try to get your own picture of it rather than thinking of how severe it is.

If you can do that, then you can modify it and you can reduce its level. For example, if you have a pain in your back like a tight band, or a taut rope, then close your eyes and visualise that rope with a great big tight knot in it. Focus hard and mentally try to loosen the knot.

You may feel that your pain is burning like a smouldering rope. Hold that picture in your mind, and imagine it getting less intense, less burning as it is soaked in water, until it is totally extinguished.

Use your imagination to remedy whatever picture your mind conjures up. A cold pain like an icicle could be warmed up and melted by imagining it being gently heated. A boring pain like a corkscrew could be gently unwound from a cork.

Sit or lie down and make yourself as comfortable as you can in a place where you will not be disturbed. Let your mind throw up images that seem right, and when you have the image that corresponds best with the pain, use your mind to reverse the effect. As you do this, tell yourself that you are reducing it, lessening the discomfort, until it goes.

Your imagination is very powerful. It can make you feel emotional, so it makes perfect sense to get it to work for you to affect the medial pain system that controls the emotional component of pain. You can use your imagination as a painkiller.

Try doing this for 20 minutes every day for a week. You may be very surprised and very pleased at the results.

15. Learn about the Life Cycle concept

I use the concept of the Life Cycle when I am working with patients. Yet this is not the life cycle that you may have learned about in biology lessons when you were studying frogs or insects. Rather, it is a way of thinking of the different components of one's life and how they each affect the other.

Imagine that there are five spheres in life, all of which are relevant to our well-being. A painful condition can affect all of them negatively. These spheres are:

Body – the physical symptoms, e.g. back pain, limited mobility, stiffness.

Emotions – how you feel generally, and how the physical symptoms make you feel, e.g. angry, sad, anxious, jealous, guilty.

Thoughts – what thoughts do you have, e.g. pessimistic thoughts, negative thoughts, self-critical thoughts, and so on.

Behaviour – how the above spheres make you behave, e.g. do you isolate yourself by avoiding things or people? Do you develop habits like smoking and drinking, or do you take too many painkillers? Do you rest and become inactive?

Lifestyle – how does your condition affect your ability to do things, or affect your relationships? Also how do events in your life impact on you?

Try drawing these out on paper, as in the following diagram:

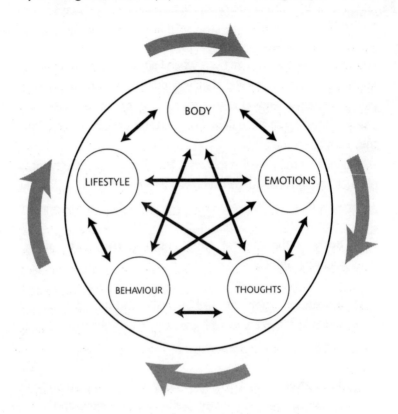

Start with Body and put it in a circle at the top of the paper. Then draw an arrow and a circle for Emotions below and to the right. Then put Thoughts below that, so that each takes up a position in a circle, or on a clock face. Thus: Body at 12 o'clock, Emotions at 2 o'clock, Thoughts at 5 o'clock, Behaviour at 7 o'clock and Lifestyle at 10 o'clock.

Now draw double-headed arrows (←→) between them, so that you can see that Body affects Emotion, and vice versa, and that each sphere in the circle can affect the ones behind and ahead.

Now draw double-headed arrows between Body and Thoughts, and between Body and Behaviour. Indeed, you will see that you can link all of the spheres up like this so that you produce an internal five pointed star. And that is the Life Cycle.

What it represents is the way that every facet of your life can affect every other part. On one hand, the Life Cycle explains how a bad physical symptom, a pain for example, can affect your emotions in a negative way. Your negative emotions can affect the way you think or the types of thoughts that you have. This in turn can make you act or behave in a particular way, which can affect your lifestyle, your relationships, and so on.

On the other hand, the Life Cycle offers you multiple opportunities to modify how your condition affects you. Essentially, a physical condition should not control you or your life. If, for example, you feel depressed because of a painful back, rather than allowing inactivity to make you worse, get active. Instead of taking to bed, get out in the garden or go into the kitchen and make lunch instead of allowing yourself to become an invalid. If your partner is taking charge, talk to them and explain that it is better if you try to do things.

Now write your experiences and ideas in each circle, recording anything that seems relevant to each category.

By recognising that you can change how you feel by doing something different in any of the other spheres of the Life Cycle you open up your list of strategies.

16. Keep a pain diary

It is worth keeping a pain diary to record your pain levels, but I suggest that you do it in connection with the concept of the Life Cycle that I have just described. Rather than just seeing what your pain level was on any one day, examine what you were doing or experiencing in the different spheres of the Life Cycle.

I suggest that you score pain on a range from nought to ten, where nought is no pain and ten is the worst pain imaginable, the pain that you would experience from being boiled in oil, perhaps.

Then mark out a series of columns running through each day. Use a column for the date, then ones for Body, Emotions, Thoughts and Behaviour. Perhaps the most useful way of recording is to note each time you are aware of a marked level of pain. If that is not convenient, then just select three times of the day and record everything then.

In the date column write date and the time of each recording. Under Body, focus on the pain and write down its level. Under Emotions record how the pain made you feel, e.g. sad, angry, anxious. Under Mind write down what you thought, e.g. did you swear? Write what your thought was: Oh dear! Oh no! This is terrible! Under Behaviour, write down what you were doing at the time, e.g. exercising, gardening, working on the computer, and then what you did about it, e.g. nothing, took a painkiller, made a cup of coffee, had a massage from your partner, and so on. You can then score your pain level after you took that action.

If you keep doing this diary then after a week or so you may see if a pattern has developed. You will see if certain things worsen or provoke your pain, and you may see which behaviour or action could improve it.

The aim is to use the Life Cycle approach to see what you did to help, or what you could have done to help. Using a strategy such as this may enable you to modify your pain levels and be able to rationalise your use of painkillers.

31 Jan '16

Chapter 4

Improve Your Posture

When you were a youngster did your parents or your teacher ever exhort you to sit or stand up straight, stop slouching or to straighten those shoulders? Most people can empathise with that. Then you grow up, do as you please and before you know it your posture is all out of balance.

Well, that may be the case, but it may also be that you just fall into certain postural habits. A lot can be down to the type of chairs and seats you have at home and at work, or the position you drive in. It can relate to your feet, how you stand, what sort of shoes you wear and how good your balance is.

The point is that if you end up with a poor posture you are liable to suffer as a result. Poor posture is one of the most common reasons for having back pain.

As I have indicated above, there are lots of factors that can result in a postural problem and we shall consider some of them in this chapter. First, I would like you to check your posture.

17. Look in the mirror

Do you use a mirror a lot? Most people use them to wash, do their hair, or check how their clothes look. But do you ever look at your posture? Possibly not. At any rate, you probably don't really scrutinise how you hold yourself. Let us change that. You need a good full-length mirror.

To get the most out of this it is an idea to strip down to your underwear, so close the door first and feel comfortable.

Stand in front of the mirror and without trying to alter your posture, just adopt your usual pose. It is the position that your body naturally falls into that you need to observe, not how you think you should try to look.

Here is what to check:

Front view (you can do this easily yourself)

- Compare both sides for symmetry.

- Are your ears at the same level?

- Is your head on one side? Your nose should be in the same line as your umbilicus (tummy button).

- Are your shoulders level? Are they the same shape or does one dip down?

- Is the gap between your arms and your torso the same? If not is there a twist to the side in your torso? If you have a scoliosis, a bend in the spine as you look straight ahead, then you will curve in on one side and bulge out on the other.

○ Are your nipples at the same level?

○ Are your hips at the same level? If not you may find that you are twisted slightly so that one side is further forward that the other. This would be reflected in your umbilicus pointing to one side rather than straight ahead.

○ Are your knees pointing directly straight ahead? Are your legs straight or they bowed outward or inward?

○ Are your feet in good shape? Look at the arches. Are they good, high arches or are they tending to collapse? If they are collapsing then the foot will tend to turn in on itself and this throws the posture out. This turning in of the foot is a natural process called pronation. I will return to it Action 21.

Side view

You may need to use a second mirror and angle it to see yourself in the main mirror, or ask someone to help you. Perhaps even get them to take a photograph of you in profile.

○ Is your head perpendicular, not pointing back or forward?

○ Are your ears and shoulders in the same line?

○ Is the bottom of your chin parallel with the floor? Ideally there should not be an angle.

◑ Is the stomach flat? It should be ideally, but if you are overweight, then a 'belly' may pull you forward, which is bad for the posture and bad for the back.

◑ Can you see the three curves? A healthy back has three natural curves: a slight forward curve in the neck (cervical curve), a slight backward curve in the upper back (thoracic curve), and a slight forward curve in the low back (lumbar curve). A forward curve is called a lordosis and a backward curve is called a kyphosis. Good posture actually means keeping these three curves in balanced alignment.

18. Nurture your three curves

Apart from looking in the mirror you can check the three curves of your spine quite easily. Stand with your back to a wall, heels about three inches from the wall. Place one hand behind your neck, with the back of the hand against the wall, and the other hand behind your lower back with the palm against the wall. If there is excessive space between your back and the wall, such that you can easily move your hands forward and back more than one inch, some adjustment in your posture may be necessary to restore the normal curves of your spine.

Having awareness of your posture and in what way it seems to be out of balance is important. It is your starting point. You will not be able to correct it overnight, nor yet perhaps in days or weeks, but if you work at it steadily then you will reap the rewards, and that means that you will have a stronger back that causes you fewer problems.

It is a good idea to check yourself in the mirror at the start of the day and at the end of the day, looking at how your posture is shaping up. And do the wall test and check on those precious three curves. Get those right, keep as symmetrical as possible and your posture will improve.

19. Stand correctly

You might scoff at this and think that you know how to stand. After all, you do it naturally, don't you? But do you do it correctly? Could that be part of the reason that you have back pain?

The fact is that standing is not good for the back. Unfortunately, it is not something that you can easily avoid since you have to stand when queuing, chatting to people in the street, using shops, banks, and so on.

What happens when you stand for too long is that the back muscles get tired and start to relax. This causes the lumbar lordosis, where the forward curve becomes exaggerated. This is actually a reverse of the problem that one gets from sitting too long (which I will come to in the next section). To ease it you need to stand more efficiently. Good standing posture lessens the risk of back pain.

You will have a good idea of how you should stand already, just from reading about how your posture should be. To stand correctly try to do the following:

1. Hold your head up straight. Do not tilt your head forward, backward or sideways.

2. Try to keep your ears in line with the middle of your shoulders.

3. Keep your shoulder blades back.

4. Keep your chest forward.

5. Tuck your stomach in and tighten your buttocks slightly.

6. Keep your knees very slightly bent; don't lock them. Locking your knees encourages the stomach to protrude.

7. Be aware of the top of your head. Imagine that you are trying to stretch it towards the sky or the ceiling.

8. The arches in your feet should be supported. I will return to this soon in Action 21.

Of course, if you have to stand for longer than is comfortable, even with a good standing posture, your back will start to experience discomfort. Even super-fit soldiers standing on parade can be subject to back pain and they are advised to make certain adjustments in how they stand to ease the pressure.

Basically you should avoid standing in the same position for a long time. Shifting your weight from side to side will help. Don't sway around like a willow tree, but transfer your weight back and forth from one foot to the other.

It is a good idea to try to elevate one foot by resting it on a stool or box, or if by a fireside, place one foot on the hearth. Then after a few minutes, swap over.

If you are working at a sink, then be careful of standing and stooping forward. This is bad for the back. Instead, bend the knees slightly forward so that they are pressing on the cupboard door beneath the sink. This will straighten the lordosis. You may also find that, while working in the kitchen, opening the cabinet under the sink and resting one foot on the inside will help. Again, change feet every 5 to 15 minutes.

20. Sit properly

Sitting is one of our main activities. Or rather, it is one of our main inactivities! And more people are doing it more often, thanks to the increasingly sedentary lifestyle that comes with the use of electronics and computing in the home and the workplace. Nowadays it is not even necessary for people to travel to work, since many jobs can be done in the comfort of one's own home. One can communicate instantly with people virtually anywhere in the world, access information any time of the day or night, and all from one's chair.

That is not a diatribe about electronics or computers. I use them extensively myself. It is simply an observation that people are, in general, less active than they were even ten years ago. More than half of the population sit for over 70 per cent of their waking life. One must ask the question, 'Is this good for one's general health, and more specifically for one's spine?'

General posture

The answer is 'no' to both parts of the question above. When you are sitting you are not challenging your system physiologically. You are putting your body into a position that does not permit for efficient breathing, for one thing. You don't move your chest to inflate the rib cage and the position of sitting, especially if you sit slouched, means that you don't use your diaphragm as much as you could. It is effective enough for the activity of sitting when you are not expending much energy, but it is not enough to keep your system as oxygenated as it should be. That is partly why one can feel sleepy and tired just from long periods of sitting.

When you are sitting you are not using as many muscles as when you are moving or standing. In particular you are not using your soleus muscle. This is a very important muscle situated deep in the calf of each leg. Referred to as the 'soleus pump', it has a very important function in returning blood to the heart. In order to make this work you have to be moving, that is, walking about. This pumps blood back to the heart more effectively. When it is not in operation, there is a tendency for fluid to come out of the circulation and to collect in the dependent soft tissues of the feet and ankles, causing them to swell. You will notice this particularly on long air travel journeys, since this lack of soleus pump action is part of the cause.

The back

With regard to the spine, sitting tends to make you lose the three curves, replacing them with one big C curve, or kyphosis. And different types of seat cause different types of C. The worst is the slouching that happens in most modern 'comfy' sofas. Their shape does not keep one upright, but tends to encourage the C shape. More than that, you end up bearing your weight on parts of the back not designed to do so, producing pressure and strain on the whole back after a while.

There is no such thing as an ideal sitting position

You will remember being castigated as a child for not sitting up properly with a straight back. It was good advice, albeit difficult to do. One of the problems is that we tend to be given desks and tables to suit all sizes. People adopt ways that seem to be comfortable for them, or which permit them to do whatever work they need to do while sitting at a desk or facing a computer.

A survey of office workers by ergonomic specialists Etienne Grandjean and Ulrich Burandt showed that a little over 50 per cent sit in the middle of the chair, 33 per cent sit back in the chair and 15 per cent sit on the front of the chair.

The sitting position depends on the design of the seat, the nature of the task being performed, the availability of the things needed for the task (how the desk is arranged, for example) and the preference of the person.

The old adage was that you had to have an upright position, with hips at ninety degrees to the spine, the shoulders back and the head as upright as possible. If you are a desk worker you may say that this just isn't feasible. There are so many things to do that you need to keep altering your posture. Certainly if you are bobbing your head up and down from a keyboard to a screen, or from a notepad or book, while you acrobatically balance a phone in the crook between your shoulder and your chin, you will know the difficulty of keeping a straight back.

What you do need to try to do is to keep the spine as upright as possible. Use the chair to give you some support in the small of the back so that you encourage that lumbar lordosis and work against the big C curve. Perhaps have a firm pad or cushion there.

The 90 degrees at the hips is hard to maintain and it is not actually a natural position for comfort. Most people sleep with their hips at about 45 degrees. That takes strain off the hips and the spine and is a good angle to aim for.

Avoid crossing your legs

This really is worth working at. Why we do it is quite odd, because it is not comfortable and it is not natural. It is learned. If you cross your legs then you are twisting the pelvis and that demands twisting of the spine to compensate. This is especially the case if you are working at a desk.

Choose your chair

You may think that being upright demands that you go for a minimalist type of chair with a straight perpendicular back. Well, that won't do much to encourage your natural curves. The ideal is one with a gentle backward curve, which will encourage the lumbar lordosis.

21. Wear sensible shoes and perhaps see a podiatrist

This might make you cringe! To some people fashion is everything. Yet I would be failing in my duty to your back if I did not suggest that you need to make sure that your shoes are not predisposing you to back pain, or even causing it.

Pronation

This is the name given to the natural inward roll of the foot as the arch of the foot collapses during walking. This occurs between touching down with the heel and lifting off with the toes, and it is a natural shock absorption. It is not 100 per cent effective, however, and some of the shock of each step will be transmitted up the legs to the pelvis and thence to the spine.

Both under-pronation and over-pronation can cause problems.

Under-pronators do not have enough roll, so they do not effectively shock-absorb. They usually have high arches and as a result they may get knee pain and low back pain. They need flexible shoes with good cushioning.

Over-pronators have too much roll and the foot collapses on each step. They get strain on the whole of the lower body and may have persistent low back pain. They generally have fairly flat arches and need some sort of support in their shoes. A medial arch support can be inserted into the shoe which may help over-pronation.

Get help selecting shoes

This is very sensible and it is worth going to shops where you will be served by someone with knowledge about shoe fitting. It may cost more, but it will be worth the investment. You need to have shoes that will be the right size for both feet, with adequate room for the toes (but not too much) and with the proper type of support. They should also be the right shape for your feet.

Never wear other people's shoes. For one thing, they will probably have become worn to their shape, so will slightly affect the way that you walk.

Heels

This is an area of particular importance. High heels may look stylish; they may give you added height and shape the calves; but they throw your posture out and definitely predispose you to back strain. A sensible heel is one of an inch and a half or less.

People who want to wear high heels (anything over an inch and a half) would be sensible to restrict their use to special occasions such as going out. High heels should be avoided if a lot of walking is going to be done.

When going out to do a lot of pavement walking, a flat shoe with good support is the right type of footwear. Any longer walking across rough terrain really demands a proper walking trainer or preferably a walking boot.

Negative heel technology shoes

Some back specialists advocate these. They are shoes designed so that the toes are actually slightly higher than the heels, usually by about 3.7 degrees. This redistributes the weight over the heel and alters the overall posture. It does take some adjustment in order to get used to them and some people experience slight discomfort for a couple of days. But thereafter they do seem to help.

See a podiatrist

If you think that your feet are causing you problems in themselves, then a visit to a podiatrist is a good idea. If you think that you may have a problem with either type of pronation, a podiatrist can do an assessment and recommend appropriate orthotics (aids or support to the foot) or footwear, or even make appropriate orthotics for you.

22. Only carry what you need

Back pain is affecting people at younger and younger ages. Indeed, currently up to 60 per cent of youngsters will experience some back pain by the age of 18 years, according to the British Chiropractic Association. This really is something that should and could be prevented.

One of the main factors is the amount of things that young people carry on their backs. It is recommended that a child or youngster should never carry more than 10 to 15 per cent of their body weight in their schoolbag or backpack. The thing is that kids, being kids, tend to accumulate more and more as the week goes on. And that is where parents need to be involved. They should at least encourage their youngsters to clean out their bag at night and only pack what is necessary for the next day. In fact, a study carried out in Texas in 2003 and published in the *Archives of Diseases in Childhood*, showed that 96 per cent of parents don't check their children's bags.

But of course, the same is true for everyone, not just young people. You should only carry what you really need, and you should carry it in the best way. I am referring here to bags that we carry. If you regularly carry a shoulder bag or use a handbag or briefcase, do you always carry it on the same shoulder or on the same side? Do you check that you only have what you need in it? I know that I used to allow my medical bag to gradually grow in weight as I added different instruments, extra books and things that I might need when I visited a particular patient. The trouble was that I often didn't empty it afterwards and it grew gradually heavier and heavier.

Backpacks are probably the best type of bag to carry your things in, since they distribute the weight evenly on both sides.

It is worth weighing any bag or backpack that you regularly carry. You may be very surprised to find that you are carrying a great deal around every day. Do you really need all that? Be ruthless, just take what you need and spare your back.

On the same subject, do you have keys attached to a belt, a mobile phone clipped to your waistband, a wallet or pocket book in a back pocket? Think about these and consider whether they dig into you when you sit down or lie back. If they do then there is a good chance that they will cause your body to get into the position of least discomfort. That may mean that they alter your posture, possibly increasing the risk to your back.

23. Don't get used to wearing a lumbar corset or using a stick

Many people wear lumbar corsets. These can be very useful if you have a painful back, since they will help to buttress the abdominal muscles and help to restrict the movement of the lumbar spine. However, they should only be used for a very short time, in my opinion only while the pain lasts, since it does not take long to get used to them. The problem is that if you are not using your own muscles, they get weaker through that disuse, with the result that you ultimately aggravate one of the causes of the back pain.

Similarly, walking sticks should only be used if absolutely necessary and only while you have the pain. They can be very useful in helping you to stay upright and counter an imbalance, but the same principle applies: if you use sticks instead of using your muscles, they are counter-productive in the long run.

But if you do need one...

If you have an underlying problem like arthritis that is causing your back problem then a walking stick may be quite helpful. In this case, make sure it is one right for the purpose and not one that you inherited from your grandfather. A standard wooden walking stick or cane has a curved handle, which is useful for hooking onto one's arm to free you to do some manual task, while lightweight aluminium ones are more robust and their length can be adjusted.

A Fischer handle is a specially moulded plastic handle which may be best for someone affected by arthritis of the hands if they have difficulty gripping.

The length is crucial. As a rule of thumb a suitably sized stick is one whose length from the top of the handle to the tip is the same as the distance from the wrist crease to the floor. Thus, when standing erect in everyday shoes, holding the stick still, the elbow will bend to about 15 degrees. This allows good extension of the stick when walking and will help in weight bearing.

Always make sure that the stick has a good rubber ferrule which will give a good grip.

Finally, use the stick the right way. If you have an arthritic hip, use the stick on the opposite side, otherwise you will just hobble and not achieve the ease that you need.

If at all in doubt about how to choose or use a walking stick, your GP can refer you to your local occupational therapist or physiotherapist for advice.

24. Make an effort to be ambidextrous

Handedness is the name given to the distribution of fine motor skills between the right and left hands. It is estimated that the vast majority of people in the world are right handed, in that they tend to use that hand for most tasks. Left handedness is much less common, occurring in 8 to 15 per cent of the population. Mixed handedness, or cross dominance, occurs when people, say, use one hand to write, yet use the other hand to throw. Ambidexterity, the ability to do any task equally well with both sides, is really quite rare, although it can be learned. Leonardo da Vinci, Michelangelo and Einstein were all ambidextrous.

The fact that people choose to maintain their handedness can have an effect on posture. Understandably, there is a tendency for the muscles of the dominant hand and arm to become better developed and markedly stronger. When this handedness is extreme it can result in the muscles of the dominant side becoming generally stronger so that they can overpower those on the other side. This can result in postural twists, inequality in the level of limbs and all the features we looked at in the mirror test. In other words your handedness can be partly responsible for postural imbalance.

It makes sense to try to balance yourself and to get the muscles on both sides of your body as strong and as equal as possible. And that means trying to become ambidextrous.

Training yourself to become ambidextrous takes time and effort, but I do think it is worth it. Not only will you become more dextrous, but you will start using muscles on the other side of the body without really being aware of it – and that can only help your overall posture.

To begin, start doing simple things like picking things up with your non-dominant hand. Use that hand to stir cups, to unscrew lids, to butter bread and so on. Then try writing and drawing with the non-dominant hand. The results may be dire at first, but gradually you will improve.

Be aware also of how you walk. Do you initiate movements with your dominant side? If so, try consciously doing it the other way.

When you dress, don't put your clothes on the same way every time; experiment and aim to use your other side. Brush your teeth, comb your hair, put on spectacles with your non-dominant hand. There is no end to the daily tasks that you can start doing with the other side.

If you are really keen and find that things are going well, have a go at juggling. Juggling is a really good skill that helps your balance. Gradually, the awkwardness will go and you will have discovered a skill that will spin over to improve your posture.

25. Try the Alexander technique or take up yoga or t'ai chi

Yoga and the Alexander technique are both worth considering as things to incorporate into your life. Both are extremely good for posture improvement and will, therefore, help you to manage back pain.

Before taking up any new form of exercise, you should consult your doctor in the first instance in order to make sure that there is nothing that you should avoid doing. For example, if you have had a prolapsed intervertebral disc, a bulging disc or nerve root irritation in the neck or of the sciatic nerve it is vital that you know whether you have to avoid any excessive bending positions.

Yoga

There are different branches of yoga, some being more meditational and spiritual, while others (such as hatha yoga) are more physical and aim to teach you how to stretch, relax and get into particular postures.

You are advised to take yoga classes under the supervision of a qualified yoga teacher, rather than try to teach yourself from a book or a video. Tell your teacher exactly what your problem is, together with any advice that your doctor has given you. That way the teacher can gauge what your personal needs are and advise you about the sort of class you should attend.

A research study in 2005 published in the *Annals of Internal Medicine* was done on a group of 101 patients between the age of 20 and 64 years, who had visited their doctor and been diagnosed with chronic low back pain. They were then assigned to one of three groups for 12 weeks, during which time they were asked to take no drugs or any treatment other than what they were being offered. One third were given weekly yoga lessons, one third had weekly aerobic exercising and the last third was a control group who were simply given a book about back pain. Their progress was followed for six months. It was found that over three to six months yoga was more effective than aerobic exercise and education (just reading the book) in improving both pain and function in patients with chronic low back pain.

Overall posture can be improved. Yoga is known to be able to improve scoliosis (lateral curving of the spine), kyphosis and lordosis. Indeed, another recent study in 2009 from the University of California and published in the *Journal of the American Geriatrics Society* found that when a group of elderly people did yoga for six months they saw a decrease in the upper spine curve of five per cent, as opposed to no change in those who did no yoga. Effectively, it reduced the excessive curve that results in the 'dowager's hump' that is so commonly seen in people with osteoporosis.

Alexander technique

The Alexander technique is a system of postural awareness that aims to make the individual more conscious of the way they use their body. It is named after F. Matthias Alexander who devised the technique to improve breathing problems he had, which had interfered with his aspirations to be a Shakespearean actor.

An Alexander teacher will demonstrate, explain and help the individual to understand how to improve their balance, coordination and function.

As with yoga, it is advisable to see your doctor beforehand in order to know of anything that needs to be avoided. Then, having gained access to an Alexander teacher, explain your condition and any restrictions that it may place upon you. Together, you and your Alexander teacher will work out how best to improve your posture, balance and general well-being. It will almost certainly help you to manage your back pain.

T'ai chi

T'ai chi is an ancient form of Chinese martial art that has been practised in the East for over seven hundred years. It is said that a monk developed it as an effortless style of combat which would allow a warrior to fight effectively, but without exhaustion. The concept came to him while watching a crane attempt to unsuccessfully kill a snake. The snake gracefully avoided its attacker with minimal effort, thereby overcoming what should have been a more powerful foe.

T'ai chi is increasing in popularity in the West, and although it was developed from a martial art, it is generally non-combative, and most people practise it without making contact with anyone else. It is said to work by encouraging the flow of energy through natural channels in the body. It also aims to help the individual to relax mentally and de-stress the system.

In t'ai chi classes, the individual learns various slow, controlled movements, involving both sides of the body, which improve posture by toning muscles as one goes through these movements. Gradually, as one becomes more adept, ever more complex movements may be learned, thereby helping to keep the body both toned and supple.

Like yoga and the Alexander technique, it is most effective when it is taught by a qualified instructor.

Chapter 5

Benefit From Movement and Exercise

It may surprise you, but unless you are a tortoise or a sloth, you are designed to move and to move regularly. Inactivity is positively bad for the back. We looked at it in Action 7, Rest for a short period only, since bed rest was advocated in the past. Nowadays inactivity is discouraged, unless you have a serious fracture of the neck or the spine. But even then mobilisation is needed as soon as possible.

In this chapter I am going to talk about different types of exercise that you can do. It is not just about keeping fit and trying to maintain muscle tone. There are different types of exercise that you can do to achieve different things. And each, in their own way, will contribute to your overall ability to manage your back problem.

26. Keep on the move to prevent stiffness

The more you are moving about the better. Inactivity leads to muscle weakness, which leads to less stability and will effectively worsen the problem. It also leads to stiffness. This can be stiffness in the joints, the muscles and the tendons that join the muscles to the bones.

Thixotropy

Thixotropy is the property that some gels or fluids have of becoming less viscous, less thick, when they are agitated or subjected to a shearing force. Upon standing they can return to their original viscosity. If you think of toothpaste in a tube, it is a gel inside the tube, but when you compress the sides, it turns into a semi-fluid and oozes out of the tube, then resets immediately on the toothbrush.

You may wonder what relevance this has to back pain. Well, the fluid inside muscle fibrils, the actual muscle cells, is thixotropic. It is semi-liquid, like the toothpaste as it is squeezed out of its tube, when it is in action. But when it is inactive, it becomes more viscous and gel-like.

The same thing happens with joints and with tendons. This is partly why you feel stiff first thing in the morning. It is not simply that the muscles have become used to being inactive after a sleep, it is because there has been a change in the viscosity of the fluid within them.

When you are in pain you may feel that movements make the pain worse, and therefore you tend not to move as much. This is not the best course of action, however, since the more you keep moving the more your body will become used to the movements and the pain level will actually drop. Certainly you will be less stiff if you move.

Understandably, people worry in case extra movement during pain will worsen matters. In the vast majority of cases of chronic back pain the extra movement will only help you.

However, if the back pain is from an inflammatory arthritic condition, such as rheumatoid arthritis, then the basic principle is not to try to work through pain, as this can damage the joints if they are acutely inflamed. Having said this, rheumatoid arthritis does not tend to occur chiefly in the back.

It is important to have a diagnosis in the first instance, as mentioned in Action 6, Visit your GP, in Chapter 1. If you do have rheumatoid arthritis, then check with your own doctor about which activities are suitable for you.

Osteoarthritis, the usual 'wear and tear' arthritis of ageing, is another matter. It is important to keep moving if you have it, since movement helps to reduce stiffness.

27. Exercise to reduce pain

Exercising to reduce pain is all about improving posture and being aware of the positions that your body gets into, the positions that the body has adopted in order to experience least discomfort.

Imagine that you have a problem with your neck, for example. There is inflammation and pressure on a nerve from the neck as it comes out of the cervical vertebrae. The body then does what it can to reduce that pressure. It may drop the shoulder to take the pressure off the nerve. But it does this by contracting a segment of muscle that moves the cervical spine slightly. It will then go into spasm to maintain that position. The effect of this is twofold. First, it automatically limits movement of that part of the body. Second, after a while the prolonged state of contraction or spasm of the muscle will send out a cramp signal and pain will be perceived. Thus, pain and limitation of function will be the end product.

The simple exercises I suggest here are intended to ease the pain and release the affected muscles directly. They are exercises done using other muscles which will help the body to get into better posture and so naturally help the contracted 'spasmed' muscles to relax. That will result in the release of pain and improvement in function. The effect of doing these exercises can be quite dramatic.

Here are some simple exercises to try when you are experiencing discomfort in your back:

Sitting knee squeeze

For this you need an upright chair and a firm cushion. Sit on the chair with your feet flat on the floor at 90 degrees to your shins, so that your knees are bent at ninety degrees. Sit upright so that your whole trunk is at ninety degrees to your thighs and try to sit as tall as possible, as if you are trying to push the top of your head towards the ceiling. This is the position that encourages the three curves of the spine.

Now put the cushion between your knees. Slowly squeeze and then slowly relax your thighs so that you clasp and unclasp the cushion. Do this a dozen times, and then rest. Do three sets of a dozen repetitions.

Gradually, you will tone and build the adductors of the hips. These are muscles which stabilise the hips. This will help the pelvis to move better and in turn this will cause unlocking of the spine so that you start to get your three curves back. When this happens, your pain will definitely improve.

Lying knee squeeze

If you think of what you would look like if you tipped the chair over so that you were lying on your back, that is the position for this exercise. But please do not try to tip backwards for this; you do not want to injure your back or head!

For this exercise you need the chair or a footstool or a stack of firm cushions (the chair should be the right way up, by the way!). You need to lie on your back on the floor and place your calves on the chair or stack of cushions, at a height so that your thighs are at right angles to your back, and your shins are at right angles to your thighs. Essentially, you should have 90-degree angles at the hips and at the knees.

In this position again place the cushion between your knees and slowly squeeze and then slowly relax your thigh muscles as you clasp the cushion. Do this a dozen times. Do three sets of a dozen repetitions. Try arching your back ever so slightly during this. If you have a lot of spasm, your back may not let you arch it at first, but keep trying.

This again tones the adductors, but removes gravity, and it will help the pelvis to release, in turn helping the spine to become freer.

Alternate lying knee bend

For this you adopt the same position as in the last exercise, but only for one leg; the other rests flat on the floor. (You will need to move the chair or other support to one side in order to stretch one leg out flat.) Stay in this position for ten minutes, and then swap over for ten minutes on the other side. This exercise is also good for allowing the pelvis to become freer and, as a result, it eases the back.

Knee hugging

When you can do the last exercise easily and comfortably, try doing this without the chair or the cushions. With one leg flat on the floor, bend your other leg at the knee as much as you can, and throw your arms about the lower leg so you can hug it round the knee. Try to bring your thigh down towards you so that it touches your trunk. Hold that position for just five seconds at a time. Do the same with the other leg, and repeat five times on each side.

This exercise is great for improving lower back flexibility.

Face-down shoulder release

You need two cushions for this. Place the cushions on the floor and lie face downwards between them, with the cushions at shoulder level. Then lay your arms over the cushions so that your shoulders are slightly stretched upwards. Make a 'thumbs up' sign with each hand and point the thumbs towards the ceiling.

This helps to release the shoulders, which in turn will relax the back muscles. As a result, you will not feel so hunched up.

Gentle spinal rotation

Stand with your feet about six inches apart. With your arms stretched out in front of you, gradually turn your trunk as far as you find comfortable. Do this one way then the other, so that you build up a rhythm. Continue this exercise for 30 seconds.

Aim to go through this whole routine somewhere warm (never do it in the cold, as this is bad for the back), once a day. There are many more exercises that can be added to this, but I have found that this simple regime works well, is easy to do, and brings positive results.

28. Exercise to strengthen the back

The principle here is that you should not try too hard too soon. If you have a back problem then you have to adopt the softly, softly approach. You have to gradually build up your exercise regime and not think that you can suddenly make your back stronger. Go slowly and steadily and you will get there.

The difference between this sort of exercise and the last is that this has to be more aerobic, whereas the last was mainly about stretching. These exercises are about building strength, so that your muscles will support the back better.

Strengthen your back with a little light exercise every day

Many people with back problems have a tendency to wrap themselves in cotton wool and never risk hurting their back again. This is counter-productive as I have indicated throughout this book, since the muscles have to be used or the back pain will worsen. If you don't use them they get weaker. It is as simple as that.

So vacuuming the house, gardening, sweeping, gentle digging and mowing the lawn are all good for the back. They all get you using muscles and they get you moving. What I would emphasise, however, is that you should aim at being two-sided. Don't get into a one-sided sweeping or digging pattern. Keep changing sides.

29. Exercise to strengthen your tummy

This is crucial, although most people with back problems do not do it enough. The reason for this is that they tend to be scared, because bending is perceived as being a danger, perhaps because an episode of back pain came on once while bending. The result of course is that the abdominal muscles just get weaker and before long the muscles sag and weight may be put on, all of which pulls you forward, leaving you facing a worsening situation. Sitting is also bad for the abdominal muscles since it makes them relax and sag.

The back must not be thought of as separate from the front of the body. You need your front to be strong in order to help the back to move and function correctly. Effectively, if the abdominal muscles are in good shape they will help your back muscles to give your back a good curve.

The rectus abdominis is the strong muscle that flexes the abdomen. It extends down the front of the abdomen from the lower rib cage to the top of the pelvis. This is the muscle that gives that desirable six-pack.

The oblique abdominal muscles run across the abdomen in bands at oblique angles. There are two sets: the external oblique muscles, which run diagonally to hold the abdominal cavity tight; and under this, the internal oblique muscles, which are at a slightly different angle and give further support to the abdomen. The oblique muscles are involved in bending and twisting movements of the trunk.

Strengthen your abdominal muscles with abdominal curls

Lie on your back and bend your knees so that you can place your feet flat on the ground. Now cross your arms and place each hand on the opposite shoulder. Then lift your head off the floor, looking straight up at the ceiling as you do so. Do ten of these at a time.

Do not try to lift too high until you have built this up over a few days, or even a couple of weeks. Then try lifting so that your shoulder blades are just off the floor.

You can also do an abdominal curl by clasping your hands behind your head, then lifting one knee to touch your opposite elbow. Hold for five seconds then do the other side. Do five of each.

Never do this without bending the knees.

Make this a regular exercise every day.

30. Choose sports that are good for the back

Sport is an enjoyable way of getting exercise. You do not want to risk further injury to the back, so make sure that the sports you choose are within your capability. It would be foolish, for example, to take up a combat sport after having had a prolapsed disc.

With any physical sport which involves putting the body through bends, twists or lifts, you must always warm up beforehand.

When taking up a new sport it is sensible to check with your health adviser about things that you should and should not do. Make sure that you have an idea of what the sport will involve so that you can get an informed opinion.

Two-sided sports

By this I mean sports that involve both sides of the body. These are better for the back than one-sided sports.

Walking – this is probably the very simplest and one of the best sporting activities that you can indulge in for your back.

Jogging – this is also good, but you will have more juddering impact on the back than with walking. Do be sure to build up your distance slowly, and ensure that you have adequate footwear.

Swimming – this is excellent, since it is a two-sided activity and it is not weight-bearing. The breaststroke may hyper-extend the neck, so be careful if you have a neck problem. It is good to vary your stroke. If you are a poor or mediocre swimmer, consider having improver lessons and build up your repertoire of strokes.

Rowing – this uses many muscles and is good for strength and flexibility. If you don't fancy actually getting on the water in a boat, then a rowing machine is a good substitute.

Cycling – this is also a good exercise for strength and endurance. Do make sure that you are in a good, comfortable position for the back. Once again, if you do not want to get out on the road, an exercise bike is a good substitute and will benefit the back.

One-sided sports

Here you have to be careful, since many of these activities demand that you get into a particular position or adopt a movement that will throw a strain on one side of the body. These are enjoyable, but you do need to have an awareness of your ability and be wary of injury.

Golf involves walking and striking a ball around a course, striking the ball anywhere between 72 (many courses have a par of 72) and 110 times. For most of these shots you will actually have to strike the stationary ball hard. This means that you have to perform a swing which will result in you repeating an action which will judder your spine many times in the course of a round. Many people who play golf have back problems from this one-sided hitting. That does not mean that you should avoid it; just be careful. Have lessons from a professional, but avoid repeated striking on a golf range. You are better playing on a course, walking between shots, rather than standing still and striking a hundred balls.

Racket sports such as tennis, squash and badminton all demand fast movements, rapid changes of posture and twisting. This, coupled with one-sided hitting, make them sports to be careful with, as it is easy to strain the back while playing these sports.

Pitch and contact sports

Sports such as football, hockey and rugby are all potentially hazardous for anyone with a back problem. Rugby is a contact sport and is not suitable for anyone with a back problem. Football is also a game to avoid for people with a back problem, because of the rapid twisting, stretching and kicking. Hockey is not a contact sport, but it combines the movements of football with one-sided hitting.

All combat sports are not good for the back.

Competitiveness

It is natural that people like to give their all when they play sport. To be competitive, to play to win, are for many people at the very heart of sports. The problem is that in order to win, you have to try harder and that may mean straining that bit more, twisting further than you mean to, and so on. It is not easy to pace yourself in competitive sports, and if you are competitive by nature and you have a back problem then you may be better off considering another sport where you can afford to let your competitive urge have free reign without the unnecessary risk.

Before taking up any new sport, it is worth getting advice and having a fitness program worked out with a professional fitness coach who is aware of the limitation you have with your back.

Chapter 6

Consider Adapting Your Lifestyle

If you have a back pain problem which just keeps flaring up, you really ought to examine your lifestyle and consider whether there are certain things that you do which are contributing to the flare-ups. That is, don't think that the back pain happened just because you twisted or lifted badly. It could be that there are other things that contribute to the problem, and that the twisting movement simply pulls the trigger of a gun that is already primed and loaded ready to go off.

This chapter is all about reducing your risk and also about considering some things that you can actively do to help.

31. Stop bad habits

All habits are a form of learned behaviour. We talk about some habits being 'good', in that they serve some useful purpose. For example, brushing your teeth after a meal and putting on your safety belt as soon as you get in the car are both good habits to get into. On the other hand, we talk about bad habits when they are aesthetically unpleasant, hazardous to health or liable to lead to other problems.

Smoking

This is one of the very worst things you can do in health terms. Ever since Richard Doll and Austin Bradford Hill proved the association between lung cancer and cigarette smoking in 1950 the evidence has accumulated of smoking's adverse effects on all aspects of health. Back pain is no exception.

A research study from Norway in 1996 studied 6,691 people between 16 and 66 years of age. There were equal numbers of males and females. The researchers found that those who smoked were twice as likely to report pain as those who did not smoke. The interesting thing is that the smoking history was an independent factor, meaning that it actually seemed to have an effect on pain levels in itself. It is possible that the effect of smoking is actually involved in the mechanism of pain perception. It also seems possible that it magnifies the problem, by reducing the body's ability to repair itself.

If you need help to stop smoking, your GP can arrange help with a smoking cessation clinic.

Alcohol

Sensible alcohol drinking is OK. That means no more than 21 units a week for men or 14 units for women, a unit in this sense being a small glass of wine, a pub measure of spirits or half a pint of beer. People with chronic back pain often do drink more than this, but there is a potential problem. Alcohol is a depressant, not a stimulant. Its apparent stimulatory effect after a small amount comes from the fact that it reduces the activity of inhibitory neurones in the nervous system and one's mood may seem to lift. That is a relaxing effect. When one has more than that, more neurones are inhibited, affecting movement, making speech slurred and so on. Even more can lead to disordered thinking and the disinhibited behaviour of drunkenness.

Regular heavy drinking will cause the inhibitory neurones that I mentioned first to function at a poor level. This is the depressant effect of alcohol: as well as affecting emotions, it can allow pain signals to be perceived more readily. That is, pain is felt more often and more regularly than it would be by somebody who does not drink heavily.

So, sensible and responsible drinking only is my advice.

Recreational drugs

I refer here to so-called recreational drugs, like cannabis. People sometimes claim that they get ease from back pain with cannabis. My view is that this drug is not safe and has been shown to be positively dangerous to certain people, who may experience anxiety or even have a psychotic illness precipitated by it. Added to the fact that they are illegal, I think recreational drugs should certainly be avoided on health grounds.

32. Cut out the junk food and aim for a healthy BMI

Being overweight undoubtedly predisposes you to back pain. Extra weight throws a strain on the vertebrae, the ligaments and the muscles of the trunk. Ideally you should aim for a Body Mass Index (BMI) between 18.5 and 25. Body Mass Index is an accepted means of relating weight to height. It is easily worked out by dividing the weight in kilograms by the height in metres.

If you are aiming to bring your weight down, then make it a long term goal to get to a BMI of 25, and choose slow and realistic targets on the way.

Junk food

By junk food I mean 'fast' food with added fat, sugar and salt, and processed foods with lots of additives.

The fact is that junk food tends to promote inflammation. The fats used in preparing it include trans fats and saturated fats. These promote inflammation because arachidonic acid, one of the fatty acids found in these fats, is broken down by enzymes into prostaglandins and leukotrienes. These are chemicals that are known to trigger inflammation. If you already have inflammation that is causing your back pain, then eating junk food is liable to make it worse.

Diets high in sugar have also been associated with increased inflammation, as well as predisposing you to obesity and diabetes. It is worth eliminating high-sugar foods such as fizzy drinks, pastries, pre-sweetened cereals and confectionary from your diet. This doesn't mean that you shouldn't have them as treats, just don't have them too frequently.

Check if preserved foods have nitrates in them. These are used as preservatives in a lot of processed foods, and they also promote inflammation.

Fast eating

One of the reasons that fast-food outlets do so well is because people are in a hurry. But fast eating is not good for your system. Skipping meals, eating on the move, bolting food down or eating too late are all patterns that tend to lead to problems in the long run.

All of your digestive functions are controlled by part of your nervous system, which only operates effectively when you are calm and at rest. When you are up and being busy then it practically shuts down, so that your muscles get the lion's share of oxygen. This means that the digestion is delayed until later and the food just sits there fermenting. This can lead to bloating from excess gas production and constipation.

You should aim to eat at regular times, preferably sitting at a table, having wholesome nutrient-rich, fresh food rather than processed meals with extra fat, salt and sugar. Try to get out of the habit of having a quick sandwich or, worst of all, eating on the hoof.

33. Use anti-inflammatory foods and spices

Just as junk food may promote inflammation, your diet can include foods that are anti-inflammatory.

Foods containing omega-3

These are known to reduce inflammation and it is worth using these oils instead of saturated fats in your diet.

You will find that lots of foods, like spreads, juices and even milk have added omega-3s, which is good because the average British diet is really quite deficient in omega-3s. However, it is more efficient to get the omega-3s in their natural form, that is, from oily fish, such as salmon, mackerel or sardines. Aim to have two or three portions a week. Vegetarian-friendly sources such as linseed or flax oil can also be used.

Important

Omega-3s can thin the blood and therefore should not be taken if you are on anti-coagulants or aspirin.

Three anti-inflammatory spices

I think that it is worth considering using these three spices in your cooking. They have all been shown to have anti-inflammatory properties and may help if used regularly. They are all 'heating' herbs, which means that you do you need to be careful since they can cause indigestion for some people.

Curcumin

This is the active ingredient in turmeric which gives it its vivid yellow colour. It is also used to colour mustard powder. In trials it has been found to be as effective as hydrocortisone (a steroid) as an anti-inflammatory agent. Turmeric powder can be added to rice dishes, egg salad, salad dressings, curries, beans and sauces.

Ginger

The active ingredient here is gingerol, which is a natural anti-inflammatory agent. It works by inhibiting some of the inflammatory prostaglandins, which are natural mediators of inflammation in the body. Ginger can be taken as a supplement, in a dose of 500 mg to 1,000 mg daily. Alternatively, you can use powdered ginger on desserts or in baking. You can also use fresh ginger root in many savoury dishes.

Capsaicin

This is the active ingredient in cayenne or red chilli peppers. It is definitely known to have anti-inflammatory effects when taken in food. In you enjoy chillies in your food then this may be a good way of taking a natural anti-inflammatory substance. Incidentally, capsaicin is a hydrophobic substance, which means that it dislikes water and is not dissolved by it, which explains why drinking water will not relieve a burning mouth after eating chillies. All that water does is spread it around the mouth to, paradoxically, make the burning pain worse. If you find yourself in such a situation then drink milk or a little alcohol, since capsaicin can be dissolved in fat (which milk contains) or alcohol.

Antioxidants

Antioxidants are natural chemicals that are involved in the prevention of cell damage, which is the common pathway for inflammation, ageing and a whole host of degenerative diseases. They do this by mopping up free radicals, which are the culprits that cause the problems.

In many metabolic processes where oxidation takes place, free radicals are produced. These are atoms or groups of atoms with an odd number of unpaired electrons that can start chain reactions, in the same way that rows of dominos tumble into one another. The end result is damage to cell components, such as the DNA and the cell membranes. You can think of this as being rather like leaving a rubber band exposed to the air for a long time; it becomes friable and frayed. If you think of that happening to cell membranes, the insides of vessels and the tissues of the back, then you can see how the effects can be far-reaching.

Everyone knows that you should eat five portions of fruit and vegetables a day. It sounds simple, but a lot of people never manage that much. It is worth trying to eat your five 'the colour way', by eating five pieces of different coloured fruit and veg each day. If you do that you will be taking in a healthy supply of antioxidants, which will help reduce inflammation.

Water

This is the ultimate energy drink. Staying hydrated will ensure that your system functions at its best. About 75 per cent of the population are probably slightly dehydrated most of the time.

If you simply increase your water intake to six to eight glasses of water a day (no more than that), you may significantly reduce your back pain level.

34. Consider taking supplements

If you are on any prescription medication then do check with your own doctor to make sure it is OK for you to try supplements.

The following are worth considering if your back pain is due to underlying arthritis.

Glucosamine sulphate and chondroitin sulphate tablets

These chemicals are both components of cartilage. In 2001 an important paper was published in *The Lancet* by a team from Belgium, Italy and the UK, led by Jean-Yves Reginster. They demonstrated in a three-year study that glucosamine sulphate markedly halted the progress of osteoarthritis, and that it actually halted cartilage destruction.

The effective dose of glucosamine sulphate is 1,000 to 2,000 mg daily. If it is taken on its own I usually suggest 500 mg three times a day. The effective dose of chondroitin sulphate is also 1,000 to 2,000 mg daily. When the two are taken in combination, then the lower dose of 1,000 mg for each seems to be adequate.

Allergy alert

Glucosamine sulphate is derived from shrimp, crab and lobster shells. it must not be taken by anyone who is allergic to seafood. It is best avoided by anyone who is taking an anti-coagulant or aspirin

Chondroitin sulphate is derived from pork or beef cartilage. Both glucosamine and chondroitin contain sulphate, so if you are allergic to sulphates you should avoid it.

MSM tablets or capsules

Methylsulfonylmethane, to give its full name, is a good source of sulphur. This can be a wonder supplement to people who are low in sulphur – the problem being that there is no readily available test to determine a person's sulphur level. I have found this to be very effective in people with very painful osteoarthritis and in some people with chronic back pain.

The dosage is 1,500 to 2,000 mg daily. Occasionally, people experience a worsening of symptoms for a week or two, but this is usually followed by an improvement.

Obviously, if you are allergic to sulphur or sulphates then you should avoid this supplement.

Calcium and vitamin D

I mentioned osteoporosis in Action 4, Understand the causes of back pain, in Chapter 1. It is important to do all that you can to prevent this condition. That means making sure that you have a good calcium intake in your diet – cheese, milk and other dairy products are all good sources. Oily fish are rich in vitamin D, which helps you to absorb the calcium.

In my opinion it is a good idea for all women over the age of 40 to take a daily calcium and vitamin D tablet, in order to reduce their risk of osteoporosis, but do check with your own doctor.

35. Get help at work

Where you work and what you do at work can have a direct effect on your back.

Ergonomics is the name for the study of the way that people interact with their environment. Most employers should be able to access an ergonomic assessment if you are having trouble with your back at work, so that you are not put at risk of further injury or strain.

The type of work you do

The truth of the matter is that most jobs are not designed to the individual's needs, since workers are of varying age and fitness, and have a propensity to want to do things in their own way.

Desk-based jobs – if you sit for a large part of the day, your seat and work station should be assessed ergonomically. The seat needs to be comfortable (see Action 20, Sit properly). If you are using a computer, the seating height may need to be adjusted. It is best to sit back in the chair so that you bear your weight on your pelvis, not on your thighs. A lumbar support should be incorporated into the chair design.

The arrangements of things on the desk and your computer keyboard may need consideration. It is possible to get an ergonomic keyboard which is curved to allow you to get into the right posture.

The height of the computer screen may need adjusting so that you do not end up putting too much strain on the neck. The centre of the screen should be at eye level. This is a rule of thumb, and ideally it should be assessed individually according to the worker's needs.

You should be able to get up frequently to move around, otherwise there is a tendency to slump. In addition, getting up and walking about helps by getting the soleus muscles working, which makes swelling of the ankles and feet less likely. You will remember that we discussed the 'soleus pump' effect in Action 20.

Standers – if you spend much of your working day on your feet, then look at the surface you walk or stand on. Good and appropriate footwear is essential.

Lifters – if you have to carry things in your work, or have to lift weights, then it is important that you do not have to undertake any heavy lifting that could be injurious to your back. It is imperative that you lift correctly and that there is provision for looking at this in your job.

Drivers – if you spend a large part of your working time sitting in a car driving, then you should look at your driving position. Sitting too far forward hunched over the wheel or reclining too far back with the arms outstretched to hold the wheel can both cause back problems.

Incorporate some exercise into your work

If you are sedentary, you need to be able to do something to help keep your muscles in tone. Some simple stretching at your work station or during your breaks will help. It is not something that you should feel embarrassed about asking for, since it is in everyone's interests that you are able to manage your back pain at work.

And when you get home from work

Do not slump into a chair. You may feel the need to rest after a hard day's work, but if your job has been throwing a strain on your back, the last thing you should do is slump and exacerbate the back again.

This does not mean that you should not relax, but just be aware that there are other ways of relaxing than just sitting in front of the television. And the same thing goes for laptops, home PCs and games consoles. You don't want to merely continue the same strains at work when you arrive home.

If you have been sedentary at work, then home time is good for some non-sedentary activity. Think about how you can use your time pleasurably and well, to help you manage your back better, such as gardening, cooking, taking the dog for a walk, etc.

36. Learn to lift properly

Everyone should learn how to lift properly. You might think that it is something that we do naturally, but it is not. People just learn to lift through experience after seeing other people do it. Lifting safely is not something that is taught as a matter of course (unless it is an integral part of your vocation).

Stand with feet apart – you want to give yourself a broad base to lift from. This will help with your balance. Aim at the width of your shoulders or slightly less.

Get close to the thing that you are going to lift – your intention is to lift straight up, not at an angle. If you have to lean then you are angling your back, and so are at risk of straining it.

Bend the knees – this is the one that everybody seems to know about, but which is ignored most of the time. A common reason for not bending the knees when lifting is that if you consciously think that something is not heavy you eliminate from your mind the possibility of hurting yourself. This is a mistake, because the correct lifting of all weights will prevent the unexpected. The whole aim of bending the knees is that you will be able to lever the weight upwards with a straight back.

Get a good, stable grip – people often strain their backs or injure themselves in other ways by trying to lift things in an unorthodox way. They may have several things in one hand and try to lift something one-handed, in such a way that they will have to arch their spine laterally in order to do so. Do not do this. Always use both hands, and don't try to lift several things at a time or try to save time by lifting too much at once. Finally, don't force yourself to balance things like an acrobat by lifting unstable piles of things.

Keep your weight towards your heels – when you start to lift you need to have a broad base as mentioned above, but also to keep your weight towards the heels and the outside of the feet, since this engages the core muscles. You should not try lifting when you are balancing on the balls of your feet.

Breathe out when you lift – this is very important. You should not hold your breath as many people do when they lift. You should always breathe out when making the effort. This applies whether you are lifting a kettle, a bag of cement (although you should get help to do this), making a golf swing or striking a ball with a racket. It is worth getting into the habit in your normal daily activities.

Don't try to imitate a weight-lifter – by that I mean that you need to lift smoothly, pushing upwards with your legs, so that they do all the work. You are not trying to hurl a weight above your head like a weight-lifter, so do not heave; take your time.

> ### Putting down needs thought too
>
> Essentially, you have to take good care when you put the object down as well. There is no sense in protecting yourself for the lift, only to strain yourself in the put-down. This should also be a smooth movement: a reverse version of the lift.

Things to avoid in lifting

Too large a weight – if it is made up of several things, then split it up and take smaller loads.

Pulling the load before the lift – if you can, it is always easier to push.

Twisting – this is the extra movement that tends to strain facet joints. It is that extra twist that causes many a back to 'go'.

Reaching that extra few inches – a letter falls to the ground, you bend and a breeze moves it a few inches. You have already bent, but now you stretch – and the back suddenly 'goes'!

Lifting too high – if you have to stretch your back backwards to get that extra bit of height, then you are trying to lift too high. That is a time to ask for help.

And remember: never be embarrassed to ask for help.

37. Choose the right bed

When you consider that you probably spend a third of your life in bed, it makes sense to make that time as comfortable as possible and as beneficial to your back as you can.

The position you sleep in

Do you move around a lot in bed? Some people seem to do so naturally, changing their position frequently throughout their sleep time. Some who do are dimly conscious that they do so because they do not feel comfortable. If you are in the latter category then you may find that you wake feeling stiff and with an ache in your back.

People who sleep on their back are most likely to wake feeling uncomfortable. This is because lying on the back with your legs straight out tends to throw the back into an exaggerated curve in the low back area.

The best position for the back seems to be lying on your side with the knees bent to about a 45-degree angle. Trying to get into that position is a good idea. Putting a pillow or a small cushion between the knees may make it more comfortable.

If you can't get used to lying on your side, then try using a pillow or cushion under your knees to create the knee-bend, to take some of the pressure off the lower back. People prone to sciatica usually find this helps.

People who lie on their front may find that trying to sleep on their side is helpful, because they are then more likely to get their legs into a more relaxed position as mentioned above. Lying on the front will straighten the legs.

The mattress

In days gone by people would buy one mattress and keep it for life. They believed that it wore into your shape. More likely, it becomes misshapen and your body accustoms itself to that misshapenness with an inevitable effect on the posture. Ideally, you should get a new mattress every ten years. It should, of course, be turned about once a month, but preferably by two people!

As to how firm or how soft it should be, there is no answer to fit all backs. It is partly personal preference, but soft mattresses are not good. If your mattress is too soft it is going to buckle and not give you support. Similarly, it must not be too hard, since that would be like lying on the ground. You do need some cushioning.

Modern memory mattresses are excellent, because they conform to the shape of the person's body and they adapt to any movements of the body. I use one and personally recommend them. (I hasten to add that I have no arrangements of any sort with any mattress firm or organisation!)

Pillows

You should always use a pillow or two, to allow the neck to be supported. Special neck pillows are available for those who suffer from neck pain.

Avoid bed boards

It used to be standard advice to tell people to put a board or a door under the mattress to give extra support. This is not a good idea because it will interfere with the working of the mattress and there is no good evidence that it is of any benefit.

38. Enjoy your sex life

A loving, active sex life is normal and it is a shame if a chronic back problem stops it or severely restricts it. Back pain may limit your activity, but there are still things that you can do to keep the passion going, and ways that you can pleasure each other without causing pain.

How is your libido?

This is a question to ask oneself. Back pain can make people avoid sex if they have found that the act causes more pain. Unconsciously, the libido can get turned down or switched off.

Both anxiety and depression can also reduce the libido. Anxiety about injury or anxiety about performance can diminish the desire for sex. Depression can itself reduce libido. Indeed, if you realise that your libido is reduced then it is worth considering whether depression is the problem.

If you think that you are avoiding sex because of anxiety or if you suspect that you could be depressed, then you should see your GP, since treatment of the underlying emotional problem may make a big difference. And as mentioned before, depression itself can worsen back pain.

What is your partner's libido like?

This is also worth asking, since your partner may have experienced a drop in libido themselves. If your partner is anxious about hurting you, then they may have developed anxiety or started to get depressed. And remember that anything affecting one partner will potentially affect both of you. So if it seems that the answer is yes to either of these issues, then seeing your doctor makes sense.

A sex life is not just about sex

Without wishing to get into any wider issues about the purpose of sex, it is generally the case that an active, loving sex life is good for people. It relaxes them and enhances their well-being. Anything that helps people to relax will tend to reduce pain levels and is worth aiming at for anyone with a chronic back problem.

And that brings us to the mechanics of sex.

Take a painkiller

There is no problem in this. If you anticipate that you may have pain from your love-making then a painkiller half an hour before may remove anxiety about pain.

Positions that are best for backs

In fact, there are no 'best' positions, but there are positions that are less likely to produce problems.

The reason that people with back problems experience further pain in their backs during sex is generally because of hyperflexion or excessive bending of the spine and because of sudden jerking movements. This may mean that some of the more adventurous positions may be inadvisable, and that you should aim at less vigorous sex.

With some positions you may need some propping, so using cushions or rolled-up towels may help.

The missionary position

This is one of the most common sexual positions, with the couple facing one another, one partner underneath and the other on top. If the partner underneath has the back problem then supporting the back with a rolled towel may help to get the spine into a good, comfortable position.

If the partner on the top has a back problem, then the missionary position is still generally comfortable, but it may be worth propping your partner's pelvis up on cushions so that you can kneel, which may make things easier.

Sitting
Using a chair to sit on will support the back of the seated partner with a pain, allowing the other partner to be lowered onto the seated one comfortably.

Kneeling
For a partner with a back pain it may be more comfortable to kneel and support oneself by leaning forward on a bank of cushions, allowing your partner to enter from behind.

Lying on your sides
This can be helpful in that it permits good bending of the hips, which will help the spine to get into the right position.

The main thing is to enjoy this aspect of your life. Discussing it frankly with your partner is recommended and some planning may be needed. This may even enhance the whole prospect, and some people even find that back pain can paradoxically improve their sex life simply because consideration by both partners is needed.

Chapter 7

Be Positive About Your Back

A positive mental attitude is one of the best things you can have, in my opinion. This goes for all medical conditions, but especially for chronic conditions. It really is very easy to get down in the dumps and then to start thinking that your back is never going to get better. Even worse, you can get into the state where you expect it to get worse. Believe me, this will not help, and it can become a self-fulfilling prophecy. On the other hand, the following tips can help you to get into a positive frame of mind in order to deal with your back problem.

39. Be an optimist

If you are of a pessimistic nature then you are more likely to get depressed, feel anxious, experience more pain and even have a higher risk of conditions like heart disease. You are also more likely to pick up colds and other respiratory infections.

It is thought that this is in part due to a psychoneuroimmunological (PNI) mechanism.

The term psychoneuroimmunology was first coined by Robert Ader and Nicholas Cohen at the University of Rochester in 1975, since which time a vast amount of research has been done. It refers to the growing realisation that the mind (psyche), the nervous system (neuro) and the immune system are all interconnected. Thus, stress can affect the nervous system and thence the immune system. A lot of stress can throw a strain on the whole system, so that the immune system works below par and the body can pick up an infection.

We all operate to varying degrees of immunity, and you can have positive PNI mechanisms and negative ones. A positive mechanism is seen in people who are able to delay an illness, but who may then go down with something on the first day of their holiday. A negative one is seen when some stress is immediately followed by an illness, resulting in days off sick from work.

Pessimists are more likely to operate the negative PNI mechanisms and optimists the positive ones.

Learn about logotherapy

Viktor Frankl was the founder of a system of psychiatry known as 'logotherapy'. This is sometimes referred to as the 'Third Viennese School of Psychiatry.' Sigmund Freud's psychoanalysis is accepted as being the first, and Alfred Adler's individual psychology was the second. Frankl developed his theories during stays in three World War Two concentration camps, including Auschwitz.

In his philosophy of logotherapy, Frankl established three basic beliefs: firstly, that life has meaning under all circumstances, even the most miserable ones; secondly, that our main motivation is our will to find meaning in life; and thirdly, that we have freedom to find meaning in what we do, and what we experience.

The essence of all this is that we have a choice about how we view things. One must work against a tendency to be pessimistic and to try to become an optimist. To begin with, you have to consider 'self-talk,' or the 'inner monologue'. This is the name that we give to the endless stream of thoughts that run through a person's head every day. Pessimists, who may be more prone to depression, tend to have a lot of negative automatic thought. Let me give you four examples of such negative thought.

- **Filtering** – this is where the individual filters out all the positives and sees only the negative. For example: despite a largely good day at work, the individual will focus on the single error they may have made.

- **Personalisation** – whenever something goes wrong the individual automatically assumes it is their fault.

- **Catastrophising** – the individual extrapolates all situations to the worst scenario, usually finding a reason for not doing something to prevent a supposed humiliation risk.

- **Polarisation** – the individual sees everything as one of two poles – good or bad, black or white – with nothing between.

To think positively, you have to monitor your self-talk and try to alter the negativity. For example, instead of thinking 'I can't do it because I have never done it before,' try thinking 'It's an opportunity to learn.' Or, instead of 'There is no way this will work for me,' try 'Let me try to make this work.'

With back pain it is very important to be positive, to be an optimist. Let me refer you back to Action 15, Learn about the Life Cycle concept, in Chapter 3. If you allow yourself to become pessimistic then you will get into a particular mind-set. You will affect your emotions and tend to get anxious and depressed. And this, in turn, will make you tend to adopt particular behaviour patterns. For example, if you anticipate that you are going to have a pain, you may end up taking more painkillers; and you may also end up taking them when you do not actually need them. An optimist, on the other hand, may feel that it will go away if they do something else; that is, they adopt another behaviour pattern and distract themselves which, as we have seen, can make matters easier.

40. Be independent

If you continue to consider the Life Cycle you will see what I mean here. It is very easy to allow other people to take over various tasks which will save you from putting yourself at risk of developing pain. This is good of them, but it does not always do the back pain sufferer good. Indeed, it can lock one into the Life Cycle and lock you into a behaviour pattern of continual pain. And that is often the case with someone who sees themselves as a back pain 'sufferer' rather than someone who actively manages their problem.

Let me give an example to explain what I mean: suppose the person with back pain no longer has to do their shopping or their gardening, because their partner does it for them. Effectively, the back pain 'sufferer' is being rewarded for having the back pain. There is no incentive to stop the partner doing the task for them.

This is not ideal and it is something you should not allow to happen. You need to remain as independent as possible. That does not mean that you should refuse all offers of help all the time, but you should get into the habit of questioning what help you need. Obviously if your problem is definitely so bad that you cannot do any lifting, then you need help. And if your health advisor has told you that you should not do something, then you should accept their advice. But if matters are not clear-cut, just consider: could you do part of a task? That is, instead of having the whole thing done for you, could you do it with a degree of help?

This is actually a healthier way for you and your partner or helper to react, not with blanket restrictions, but with discussion as to how you can remain as independent as possible. It is all about being optimistic and expecting that you will be able to manage, rather than lapsing into the mindset of being a 'sufferer.'

41. Don't hold grudges

Negative emotions can have the effect of keeping your system in a state of continued stress. Prolonged anger, guilt, hate, jealousy; you can almost think of these as potential inner poisons that can eat away at you and ultimately make you ill. If your back problem is the result of an accident or if you perceive it to be somebody else's fault, then you need to be wary of letting one or more of these negative emotions take hold. There is a potential danger in holding a grudge, because it can keep a chronic problem smouldering away.

The trouble is that these emotions don't make the individual feel any better, and they are far more likely to harm the person who holds them, rather than the person they are directed against.

And just as pessimism can have a negative psychoneuroimmunological (PNI) effect, so too can all of these negative emotions, especially grudges. A disproportionate number of people who have chronic pain as the result of an accident or injury hold grudges.

People tend to justify grudges. Unfortunately, the very act of justifying a negative emotion will simply reinforce it, or in a sense will allow it to fester. And 'fester' is not a bad word to describe a grudge, because it can have the same effect as an infected wound which festers away.

The best thing is to let go of a grudge. If you do that you can move on. Try the following:

- Write down your thoughts about why you feel upset. It helps to gain a perspective on what you are feeling.

- Identify the benefits of the grudge. You will probably see that the benefits are few.

- Forget about the rights and wrongs, since you want to let go, not win an argument that the other side may not even know is being fought. Don't keep going over and over it, because that just perpetuates it and keeps it in your mind.

- Don't wait for an apology, since it may not happen. There is simply no point in setting conditions, since that is just the same as trying to justify having the grudge. This is particularly the case if you have some sort of litigation going on against a company. Don't think that you will be able to get even or make them suffer. The truth is that an organisation is not the same as a person. The organisation is not going to be lying in bed worrying.

◯ Realise that the letting go may take some time, but that ultimately it will be worth it.

◯ Talk it out, with a friend or a professional. This is probably better than just talking it over with your partner or a close relative. Having a chat with someone who has a neutral perspective can help. A partner or close relative may be too close or too concerned to be dispassionate about the situation or the feeling. That can actually have the effect of reinforcing the grudge.

◯ When you are ready, try to forgive. Only then will you be able to forget.

42. Meditate

Meditation is a technique that has been used for millennia. It is essentially a method of training the mind. There are various very different methods, such as transcendental meditation, guided imagery, and mantra meditation. The most common form used in the west is mindfulness meditation.

There have been over a thousand published studies of meditation, yet it is only recently that it has become the subject of clinical study. Mindfulness meditation is used by many psychologists and it seems to be helpful in the management of pain in general.

There was a small study carried out in Pittsburgh, USA on Mindfulness meditation in the management of chronic low back pain in 2008, published in the journal *Pain*. A small group of senior citizens all over the age of 65 years were randomly allocated either to an eight-week programme of mindfulness meditation or to a control group. The meditators were taught how to meditate and did so four days a week, for about half an hour at a time. After the eight-week period and for six months afterwards (the length of the trial) the meditators significantly reduced their levels of pain.

So what is mindfulness meditation? Very simply, it is putting yourself into a state where you induce calm in the mind, a state in which you just observe your thoughts and feelings, both emotions and physical sensations, without trying to follow them through or suppress them.

You don't have to sit cross-legged and contemplate your navel. You can do it sitting in a chair. If you do it for half an hour a day, four days a week, then the mere process of doing it may well reduce any level of discomfort that you have in your back. It will also reduce stress levels and will probably reduce the amount of stiffness and muscle discomfort in your back and elsewhere.

Basic meditation

The first thing you can try is just sitting still in a comfortable upright chair in a quiet room. Dress comfortably, perhaps making an effort to get into a relaxed mood. Give yourself a mere five minutes. If you wish you can have on gentle background music. Just get used to sitting comfortably (with a good posture, of course) and emptying your mind of thoughts.

If you find that your mind cannot empty itself of thoughts, but races around planning, solving problems or going off at tangents, then try adding a distraction. The simplest thing is a candle or a pleasing picture.

Do not be judgemental about any of the thoughts, just try to observe them and then let them go. Try not to concentrate too hard.

Then let your mind be aware of how your body feels. But try to remove judgemental words. Try not to use descriptive words. Do not think in terms of awful pain, or terrible pain. Think just of discomfort. Don't focus on one feeling for more than a couple of minutes. Then, let your mind focus on another part of the body, your head perhaps, or your knees, or your feet. Just give each part a couple of minutes (and you can do it randomly). Eventually, over several sessions, your back will 'learn' that it is only getting a couple of minutes. It is no more important than your knees or your feet, or your tummy.

You may even find that you drift off to sleep. If so, great, because you will have induced a relaxation response, which is what you're aiming for.

Repetition tunes your mind and it will have a beneficial effect in reducing your level of pain.

Chapter 8

DIY Complementary Therapies

Complementary and alternative medicine, often referred to as CAM, covers a wide range of different therapies, which are not generally considered to be part of orthodox medicine. In the UK anyone can practise certain complementary therapies without any qualification. This situation is gradually changing, and most of the therapies have regulatory or governing bodies which are trying to improve standards.

CAM includes homoeopathy, acupuncture, reflexology, chiropractic, osteopathy and herbal medicine. There are many others, but I have focussed on these ones since I believe that they can be helpful to people with back problems. If you decide to seek treatment from a professional therapist in one of these disciplines then it is sensible to ask them about their qualifications and the training they have undergone.

Many orthodox doctors, myself included, also practise therapies such as acupuncture and homoeopathy. It is also worth asking any doctor who offers such treatment what training they have had in it.

43. Try acupuncture and acupressure

Acupuncture, which uses needles to treat the patient, has been practised in China for millennia. In the traditional approach it is believed that energy flows along a series of 12 paired meridians, or pathways, and two special extra meridians. Imbalance of this energy flow can be rectified by the judicious insertion and stimulation of needles at indicated points. By contrast, Western medical acupuncture is based on physiological concepts that are accepted in Western science.

The nomenclature and numbering of the points used is common to both systems.

You cannot do acupuncture on yourself, of course, but acupressure, using finger pressure on acupuncture points may be quite beneficial. This you can do yourself. You use the pressure of the tips of the forefingers on the points and you press in a gentle clockwise manner for half a minute to three minutes at a time on each side. Do this three times a day until you feel the condition ease. You will do no harm. This really is very simple; indeed much simpler than many books would have you believe.

I find that the following five points are very useful for self-treatment of acupressure for those with back pain.

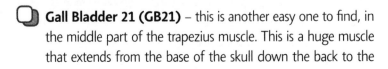 **Gall bladder 20 (GB20)** – you will find this easily, in a little hollow at the base of the skull about an inch from the midline on each side on the back of the neck. This is good for headache, neck pain and upper back pain.

Gall Bladder 21 (GB21) – this is another easy one to find, in the middle part of the trapezius muscle. This is a huge muscle that extends from the base of the skull down the back to the middle of the thoracic spine, and which spreads outwards to the scapula or shoulder blade. There is one on each side and together they resemble a large trapezoid, hence the name. If you put your hand on your opposite shoulder, the tip of the middle finger will probably be just over it. This is very good for shoulder pain, neck pain and upper back pain.

Large Intestine 4 or Colon 4 (LI 4 or Co4) – in the web between the thumb and first finger. This is a point of many uses, but is helpful if pain is severe.

Stomach 36 (St36) – in the groove between the tibia and fibula. This is good if there is sciatica or pain from the back that radiates down the legs. To find it feel just below the knee, about an inch outwards from the mid-line, and you will feel a definite groove between two bones of the shin.

Bladder 54 (B54) – this is in the crease behind the knee. To stimulate this one, lie on your back and bend your knees with your feet flat on the floor or bed. Your fingers will find it in the middle of the crease behind the knee. This is actually a really good one for easing an acute sore back.

44. Use reflexology

Reflexology is a therapy that involves a specific type of massage and manipulation of various reflex areas on the hands and feet and seems to get good results with back pain for many people. It can be self-administered to gain relief when the muscles of the back are sore and stiff, and you feel that they need a little help to relax.

The areas that are associated with the back are very easy to find and to stimulate. On the hand, this consists of the outer edge of the hand, from the wrist along the back of the thumb to the nail. The way to stimulate this is by using the tip of the thumb; press it into the side of the hand and 'walk' it, by pushing it in so that you bend the joint then advance it by straightening it out, then press, bend, then straighten – just like a caterpillar. Go up the edge several times like this on each hand.

On the feet, the area of the back is associated with the inner arch. The easiest method for stimulating this is to sit and take off shoes and socks or tights. Get a cylinder, perhaps a can of beans or an old rolling pin, and put it on the floor. Now just roll it back and forth using your foot so that it stimulates the inner arch. If it is doing its job you will find that the pain will ease as you do this.

If you find that this helps then it may well be worth seeking an appointment with a professional reflexologist.

45. Try herbal remedies

Herbal remedies can be very effective, but it is best to seek the opinion of a qualified herbalist before you try them for yourself. If you do, you should also tell your doctor that you are doing so, since it is important for them to know that you are not taking anything which could interact with your usual medication. This is extremely important in the case of Chinese herbs, since some of them have been shown to be toxic to the liver and kidneys.

It is also very important to talk with your doctor if you are considering taking anything like St John's Wort (hypericum), since it can react with several orthodox medicines, including warfarin, cyclosporin, oral contraceptives, anticonvulsants, digoxin, theophylline, or certain anti-HIV drugs.

The following herbs are certainly worth considering:

Aloe vera either taken as juice or as a capsule in a dose of 200 mg per day may be helpful in reducing pain, inflammation and stiffness.

Boswellia serrata or Indian frankincense, has been used in Ayurvedic medicine for many centuries. In the 1970s it was found to have anti-inflammatory properties that can help arthritis. If arthritis is the underlying cause of your back problem, then this may well help. It can be taken by mouth in a dose of 200 mg three times a day.

Nettle tea is a traditional remedy that does seem to help a good proportion of people. It is very bitter, however, and a little honey can take the edge off it. It has slight diuretic effects which can reduce uric acid and it also seems to have anti-inflammatory effects on joints. If you can manage two cups of it a day for a couple of weeks you may notice a difference.

Devil's claw is a plant native to the south of Africa. It is known to have anti-inflammatory properties and is advocated by many herbalists for back pain.

There is certainly some evidence that it works. A study from Germany examined its effectiveness in treating slight to moderate back, neck and shoulder muscle tension and pain. In a four-week long period, 31 people took 480 mg of devil's claw twice a day and 32 people took a placebo. The results showed there was a significant reduction in pain in the people taking herbal remedy.

Another study published in the journal *Rheumatology* compared a devil's claw extract with a standard anti-inflammatory tablet, called Vioxx. This drug, incidentally, is no longer available. The study lasted for six weeks and 79 patients were included in the trial with an acute exacerbation of low back pain. Devil's claw was just as effective as the anti-inflammatory drug.

Devil's claw should ideally be prescribed by a herbalist, and you should discuss it with your own doctor before taking it. It should not be taken by anyone with a history of stomach ulceration, or by anyone who is taking aspirin. It should also be avoided if you have a history of gall stones, or diabetes, since it can have an effect on blood sugar levels.

Quercetin is an extremely effective anti-oxidant that is found in apples, onions and tea. It may be the reason for the old adage 'an apple a day keeps the doctor away', since it does seem to be effective. It also seems to have anti-inflammatory effects. The very simplest way of taking this is in the form of an apple. I would therefore suggest that if you have a chronic back problem you eat an apple every day.

46. Get help with homoeopathic remedies

Homoeopathy is a gentle form of medicine based on the 'simile principle'. The word was coined by Dr Samuel Hahnemann (1755 to 1843) from the Greek words *homoios*, meaning 'similar' or 'like', and *pathos*, meaning 'suffering'. Essentially, this means that it is a therapeutic method using preparations of substances whose effects, when administered to healthy subjects, correspond to the manifestations of the disorder (the symptoms, clinical signs and pathological states) in the patient. The theory is that by using an infinitesimal amount of an agent that produces a similar effect to an illness, it will stimulate the body's self-regulating mechanisms to overcome the illness or symptom. It is a system that is practised across the world. Most of the remedies, of which there are in excess of 4,000, are referred to by their Latin names.

Critics of homoeopathy have difficulty with the dilute states of the remedies used, believing that this dilution is the defining characteristic of the method. It is not; the defining characteristic is the simile principle, as explained above. The individual's experience of the condition is of paramount importance, and the indicated treatment is the remedy which most closely matches the profile of the patient's experience of their illness.

Ten people could complain of back pain, yet each person's experience would be unique. They may well all need a different remedy, which is tailored to their symptom pattern. This is the great difficulty in doing research on this discipline, since there is no such thing as a homoeopathic painkiller or a homoeopathic anti-inflammatory tablet. The remedy treats the person, not a specific symptom or condition.

To get the most out of this method it is probably as well to see a qualified homoeopath. At a consultation the homoeopathic practitioner will go through all of your symptoms, focusing on how your pain is unique to you. Attention will be paid to the quality of the pain – whether it is an aching pain, or a shooting, burning, cutting or boring pain, whether it burns or feels cold. Similarly, the things that make the pain or stiffness better or worse will be noted; for they all have a bearing on the choice of remedy that you will be given.

Then again, if you feel that your pattern of symptoms matches one of the following remedies then you may find that you can start to ease your condition by trying it. These remedies are available from most health shops, some chemists and all homoeopathic pharmacies.

I emphasise that it is the pattern of the symptoms and the way that you feel that is more important than the name of the condition.

Arnica

This remedy is called 'the healer,' because it is often used for bruising injuries. It helps them to heal faster than normal. It is indicated when back pain is sore and aching, especially if it has started after an injury. If the individual always finds that the bed feels too hard, then Arnica might help.

Rhus tox

For burning pain and stiffness, which is better for movement, for heat (wheat bags, hot water bottle, etc) and for rubbing. Rhus tox is useful for pain that is generally worse in cold and wet weather.

Bryonia

This is almost the opposite of Rhus tox. Bryonia is indicated when back pain feels worse with movement and with moving around. For example, walking, bending or riding in a car may produce a lot of pain. The back may actually get red, hot and swollen. It will feel inflamed. Pressure seems to help, as does coldness, so that cold compresses and iced packs generally have been found to help by the individual.

Symphytum

This is prepared from comfrey, which has the old country name of 'knitbone'. It is a useful remedy after injury, rather like arnica. But symphytum is good for deeper injuries, if it seems that a bone or vertebra could have been cracked. It is useful for back pain that seems to have persisted for a long time after a back injury.

Kalmia

This remedy is useful for shooting and tearing types of pain. Typically, such a back pain will seem to wander, never being in exactly the same place. Or the pain can seem to travel from above down the back. Its quality can also change. Motion aggravates the pains.

Ledum

This remedy seems suited to people who suffer from chills who, paradoxically, find that cold applications really help. Unlike kalmia, the back pains that ledum is suggested for seem to travel upwards. It is also very good for problems of the feet and ankles. Swellings of joints look pale, unlike the bryonia picture.

Rhododendron

For back pains that are worse in cold, damp weather and especially thunderstorms. The person may have an extreme fear of storms. Often causes pains about the shoulders.

Ruta

For sudden strains to the back. This seems to work well if the individual suddenly pulls their back or strains a ligament.

Potency

There are different potencies of remedies available and the subject can get very complex. The most common potency scale is the centesimal (c), which means that each potency on the scale is prepared from a dilution of 1 in 100 of the preceding potency. The very start is from a Mother Tincture. Each dilution is accompanied by vigorous agitation to produce the next potency. A 6c is a potency that has gone through six successive potency preparations, each of which has been diluted 1 in 100 and vigorously agitated.

In general, use a low potency such as a 6c and take one tablet twice a day until it settles. Alternatively, take a 30c potency twice a day for three days and wait to see if the pain improves. The treatment can be repeated like this at two- or three-week intervals.

47. Use hydrotherapy at home

The early physicians of India, Greece and Rome all realised the healing potential of bathing. Public and private baths were considered an essential part of civilisation. It was also realised that it was not just the water that mattered but the way that it was used and the things that were added to it.

In the eighteenth and nineteenth centuries people flocked to the spas of Europe to take and to bathe in the healing waters of the great metropolitan centres. Naturopathic and hydropathic hotels and clinics attracted clientele from all over the world. Then, with the rapid development of orthodox medicine in the twentieth century, hydrotherapy began to dwindle in popularity and was gradually dropped from the therapeutic range of the modern physician. Yet gradually, the use of hydrotherapy is returning.

The remedial effects of water and bathing

There are three ways that hydrotherapy exerts a beneficial and remedial action upon the body.

The action of temperature on the skin
If the temperature at the skin surface is raised then more blood is diverted to it to help the body to lose heat. Thus, the skin becomes

flushed and red, and perspiration will follow to help to cool the skin. Accordingly, the circulation in the deeper tissues is reduced slightly. This can be helpful if there is deep inflammation, because diverting blood to the skin surface may reduce the circulation to the inflamed deep tissue.

On the other hand, applying cold to the skin surface will have a numbing effect and it will reduce blood to the skin surface. It will then go pale and will cool down and perspiration will be inhibited. It will have a tendency to increase the blood flow to the deeper tissues.

The mechanical effect of water and rubbing

Archimedes' principle states that a body will displace its own weight in water when it is immersed.

Because the human body is not so heavy in water it is easier to move. Exercise in water is therefore excellent when there is restriction of movement of part of the body.

Counter-irritation of the body with sprays and jets, such as you can get with jacuzzis, may help to stimulate skin nerves, which may help to override some of the pain impulses from deeper tissues. Rubbing the body while in water will also do this, and in addition, it will help muscles to relax.

The effect of additives to the bath

Here we are talking about the use of oils or salts to 'medicate' a bath. With some additives this may produce a counter-irritant effect, which can be useful. Others may work by a slight absorption of substances through the skin.

A medicated bath is one way of using aromatherapy oils. Although there is not a great deal of evidence to show that very much is actually absorbed through the skin, nonetheless certain oils do seem to have a relaxing and possibly even an anti-inflammatory effect on muscles.

Using the bath to help the back

A hot tepid bath (about 38 to 42 degrees Celsius) is going to be of most use. This is basically as hot as you find comfortable. Do not go hotter than that: it will not give a better effect.

You should not stay in a bath for longer than fifteen minutes. Indeed, sitting in a cooling bath may ultimately undo the benefits of a hot bath.

Medicated baths

There are two types of medicated bath that you might find useful: an aromatherapy bath and an Epsom salt bath.

Aromatherapy baths

Simply fill your bath so that you can sit back in it in comfort. Add six to eight drops of the chosen essential oil, then get in and soak in it for up to 15 minutes. Have a drink of cold water on getting out. Try the following oils:

- **Arnica or sage** – very good for relaxing a bruised sensation in the back

- **Cedarwood, camomile and lavender** – good for easing the aching from osteoarthritis

- **Juniper** – good if you have rheumatoid arthritis

Essential oils are available from any health shop.

Epsom salts bath

These famous salts are made from hydrated magnesium sulphate and are named after the spa town of Epsom, with its ancient healing salt spring. These are often very effective in easing aches and pains. They should not be used too often, however, since they will induce quite a marked perspiration afterwards and you can lose body fluids. If you are on any medication or have a problem with high blood pressure, heart or kidney disease, check with your doctor as to whether you should use them.

To make an Epsom salts bath you take 250 to 500 grams of Epsom salts (available from any chemists) and mix it with a little almond or other oil in a basin beside the bath to produce a pleasant wet sand feel.

Draw a warm-to-tepid bath to a comfortable temperature for you. Stand in the bath and, taking a couple of handfuls of the mixture, rub it over yourself, particularly as much of your back as you can reach. Do not put any on your neck or face, and avoid your private areas.

Put the rest of the mixture into the bath and stir it with your hands, then sit down and gently wash the salts off. After this, lie down and gradually add more hot water, keeping it at a comfortable temperature. You do not want it to be too hot. Stay in for up to ten minutes, then get out.

Having had your bath, shower down quickly with cooler water. Take care not to get out too quickly or you might feel a bit dizzy. Have a drink of water then prepare to go to bed. You do not want to do anything physical after an Epsom salts bath, so you ought to make it something that is done before bedtime.

Make sure that you wear bedclothes and expect to perspire. This in itself often feels good. Whether or not it is due to expelling toxins is debateable, but really I don't think it matters. What does matter is that it will induce relaxation, which will ease tired, stiff muscles and should help the back.

Sitz baths

The ancient Greeks favoured sitz baths. These are essentially hip baths, but with the feet in a separate receptacle containing water of a different temperature.

To make your own sitz bath you need a large basin which can be fitted into the foot end of your bath. Fill the bath with warm-to-tepid water so that it is comfortable for you. Then fill the basin with cold water. Get into the main bath and, once settled, put your feet in the cold basin at the foot end of the bath. Stay in for about 10 to 15 minutes, then remove your feet from the basin and take the basin out. Then get out of the bath.

This is often very good at easing an aching back. If you find it helpful, then have one when you feel the need of it, or aim at two a week.

You can of course medicate the warm water with an essential oil of your choice.

Showers

These are great for back pain and they have the advantage of being able to stand under a directed flow of hot water. Adjust the power of the spray if your shower allows it. The faster the jet the greater will be the counter-irritation effect, which may give greater relief. Showers cannot, of course, be medicated.

48. Use gravity to help your back

Gravity is, of course, part of the problem for the back in that we tend to be drawn downwards. The very act of standing will tend to throw a strain on your back; it is this concertina effect that can cause pressure on joints, ligaments and nerves, which may all be involved in your back pain. The good news is that you can use gravity to help, by letting your own weight exert a bit of traction to open up the joints and decompress the back. It may be only transiently, but that bit of relief may brighten your day and it will show you that back pain can always be eased if you know how to do it effectively.

Suspend your weight from a hanging bar

This is a very easy first aid move, provided you are strong enough to be able to suspend your weight from your arms and you have a hanging bar, or chin-up bar that you can fit inside a door frame. Do ensure that you are within the maximum weight suggested by the manufacturers and that the bar has been fitted securely.

All you have to do is reach up and get a good grip of the bar, then bend your knees and straighten your arms until you are hanging down. Don't do anything sudden, but when you are ready lift your feet from the ground so that you are hanging suspended by arms, your hands gripping the bar.

You then just hang there for as long as it is comfortable to do so. That may only be a few seconds, but that may be enough to help.

What you are doing here is allowing gravity to pull down, so that your back will tend to unwind, rather like a Chinese lantern does when it is hung up. It is usually quite relaxing, even if only for a short time.

Inversion table

Although this may be costly, it is an effective option. It is exactly what it sounds like: a table that tips up so that you can hang upside down from it. You strap your feet into it and lie down. Then it has a frame that you can operate yourself which will gently invert you. You do not have to go completely upside down; you can control how inverted you wish to be.

You can obtain these from many sports retailers, or obtain information from the website mentioned in Useful Addresses at the end of the book.

Again, the principle is that you use gravity to exert traction, this time supporting yourself by the feet instead of the arms. The benefit of this is that you can stay in that position for longer.

A study performed by a team from Newcastle University found that 70 per cent of people on a back surgery list were able to cancel their proposed surgery after using an inversion table for a period of time.

49. Apply a magnet or try wearing a copper bracelet

The ancients were aware that a lodestone, a naturally occurring piece of the mineral magnetite, could attract pieces of iron. Not only that, but if it was suspended by a thread it would mysteriously point to the north. Understandably, this was of incredible benefit as a means of navigation. The word 'lodestone' comes from Middle English, meaning 'leading stone'.

It was inevitable that such a magical stone, a gift from the divine, should be highly prized. Shamans and priests used them as healing stones and they attracted (no pun intended) great credibility for their success. All manner of ailments were said to be susceptible to the lodestone, from toothache and snakebites to back pain and the rheumatic conditions. Ever since, magnets have never been far from medicine and they have had a resurgence in popularity among celebrities and sportspeople, who use them to deal with all sorts of musculoskeletal problems. Interestingly, according to the *Journal of the American Medical Association*, global sales of magnets for health reasons amount to five billion dollars a year. One suspects that because Magnetic Resonance Imaging (MRI scanning) has become such a respected diagnostic tool and has entered common parlance, magnetism in a health sense has become unconsciously legitimised.

Despite the fact that there is little positive evidence that magnetism works in health, I have known many patients who seem to have derived improvement from using magnets. As long as you do not have a pacemaker which could conceivably be affected by a magnetic field, then there is no harm in trying magnets to help ease your back pain.

How do they work?

This is far from clear. Some therapists suggest that they work by enhancing the body's magnetic field. Others assert that they somehow improve blood flow to the area. I have seen no hard evidence to support either theory.

Back wraps

These are available from various magnet therapy companies and some health shops. They consist of a Velcro binding belt or wrap which has magnets inserted into pockets so that you can overlay the magnets on your painful areas.

Magnetic bracelets

These are sold in jewellers', gift shops and sports shops and many athletes and sportsmen swear by them. I can find no specific trial about their efficacy with back pain, but in 2004 a study was published in the *British Medical Journal*, about their use in patients with knee and hip arthritis. Researchers from the Peninsula Medical School studied 194 patients aged between 45 and 80 years of age from five general practices in Devon, who had osteoarthritis of either the knee or the hip. The patients were divided into three randomised groups and were asked to wear either a standard strength magnetic bracelet, a weak magnetic bracelet or a dummy, placebo bracelet. The trial lasted for 12 weeks, during which time they were asked to record scores on a recognised pain scoring scale.

The conclusion was that there was a recognised pain reduction in arthritis of the knee and hip when standard magnetic bracelets were worn, but that the strength of the magnet was important, needing to be 170 tesla (the SI unit of magnetic flux density) or greater; the study found that the weak bracelet group recorded similar levels of pain to the placebo group. The researchers pointed out that they were uncertain whether the response was due to specific or non-specific effects.

This trial is not conclusive, but there is at least some evidence of efficacy for the wearing of a magnetic bracelet. And as they are not terribly expensive, it may be worth trying one.

Copper bracelets

These are also worn by a great many people who feel that they help considerably. One trial was done in 1976 on 300 patients with arthritic pain, who were randomly allocated to either a placebo group, an active group or a control group. The placebo group were given non-copper bracelets which were anodised to look like copper and the active group wore copper bracelets. The control group were not given any type of bracelet.

There was a significant difference in the pain reduction reported by those who wore the copper bracelets as opposed to the people in the placebo and control groups. Curiously, there was also a tiny weight reduction in the copper bracelets, whereas there was no change in the non-copper bracelets. This implies that there may be a slight absorption of copper through the skin. Whether this was mirrored by a rise in the individual's copper levels was not recorded. I suspect that any amount of copper absorbed would have been negligible and certainly not enough to adversely affect health.

On the evidence I am unsure as to whether copper bracelets and magnets actually do a lot, but there is at least a suggestion that they might help. That being the case, you may find that it is worth a try.

Chapter 9

Who Else Could Help?

There is only one item in this chapter, but it is an important one since it concerns other avenues that you can try, which can be incorporated into your pain management plan.

There are a confusing number of different types of therapy which one can try. Some are available on the NHS, but you may have to consider going privately for others. Check with your GP as to whether he or she has available funding for such a referral.

If you are referred or decide to see someone of your own volition, then it is a good idea to ask about the qualifications they have and the training they received. Do not worry about causing offence; if the therapist is a member of a recognised organisation they should have no problem about answering your question. Remember, it is your back that you are asking them to treat, so you have a vested interest in knowing that they are qualified.

50. Consider seeing a specialist

As mentioned in Action 6, Visit your GP, in Chapter 1, your GP is probably the best first port of call to get a diagnosis and perhaps to get the ball rolling.

Physiotherapy

Your GP may refer you to a physiotherapist or to a physiotherapy department. Physiotherapy has always been part of the NHS and physiotherapists are used to treating back pain.

Physiotherapy is a profession that uses a variety of physical treatments to help people with a whole range of physical conditions. They use massage and manipulation with their hands to relieve muscle pains and stiffness and to help the circulation to various parts of the body. They also use heat, cold, electrical current, ultrasound, light treatment and hydrotherapy. Very importantly, they are experts in the use of remedial exercise, which is generally tailored to the individual's needs.

Finally, they can also supply aids or demonstrate the use of various aids to help an individual with various daily tasks. If someone has marked limitation of movement, for example, they can advise on aids to help with dressing, picking things up or even to help with mobility.

Remedial massage therapy

This is likely to be a private consultation. A remedial massage therapist will be trained in both superficial and deep tissue massage. This can be very good for muscular pain problems. Remedial massage therapists often run sports injury clinics. They are unlikely to do actual manipulation of joints.

Chiropractic

This is most probably going to be a private referral, although some GPs may have an arrangement with a chiropractor. Most chiropractors hold the qualification DC, or Doctor of Chiropractic, so they will use the title of Doctor. This is not a medical qualification, but is entirely separate and legitimate. Chiropractors are regulated by the General Chiropractic Council and since 1994 it has been illegal for anyone else to use the title of 'chiropractor'.

Chiropractic is a profession that specialises in the diagnosis, treatment and overall management of conditions that are due to problems with the joints, ligaments, tendons and nerves of the body, particularly those of the spine. Chiropractors are likely to perform an X-ray before beginning treatment.

Treatment consists of a wide range of manipulative techniques designed to improve the function of the joints, relieving pain and muscle spasm. Very often they use high-velocity thrusts, applying pressure directly on vertebrae to push them back into place. This often produces the clicking or cracking sound that is associated with manipulation.

Osteopathy

This also is liable to be a private referral, but again check with your GP. Like chiropractors, osteopaths are registered by their own professional body, the General Osteopathic Council, (GOsC) and it is illegal for anyone to call themselves an osteopath unless they are registered.

Osteopathy is a system of diagnosis and treatment for a wide range of medical conditions. It works with the structure and function of the body, and is based on the principle that the well-being of an individual depends on the skeleton, muscles, ligaments and connective tissues functioning smoothly together.

Osteopaths do not use X-rays as often as chiropractors, and although they also perform manipulative therapy they are more likely to use the limbs to produce a levered thrust.

There is undoubted similarity between chiropractic and osteopathy, yet they each maintain their own philosophy. The important thing is that they are both recognised and regulated professions.

Orthopaedic medicine

Orthopaedic medicine is a speciality of medicine which diagnoses and treats non-surgical conditions of the musculoskeletal system with a variety of manipulative techniques, such as dry needling or acupuncture, joint injections, injection of local anaesthetic or steroids, and other high-tech treatments. It is likely that X-rays and various types of scanning will be available.

Orthopaedic medicine specialists are likely to be doctors or physiotherapists. If they use the title 'orthopaedic physician' then they will be medically qualified and have postgraduate qualifications.

Osteomyology

This is the name used by a number of related therapies, which treat nerve, bone and muscle problems using a range of manipulative and massage techniques, often coupled with advice on nutrition and daily living. Practitioners are educated to degree and postgraduate level and are usually members of the Association of Osteomyology.

Other therapies

There are also other therapies which may help with back problems, including Bowen technique, Rolfing and the Dorn Method. I have no personal experience of them, so if you would wish to explore them then I advise you to contact their respective regulatory bodies.

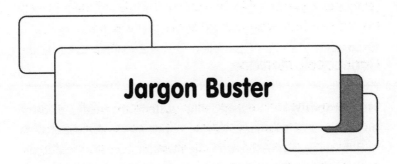

Jargon Buster

Acupressure – the use of finger pressure over acupuncture points.

Acupuncture – a treatment by professionally qualified practitioners using needles to stimulate acupuncture points.

Acute pain – normal pain from an injury or inflammation, which is usually self-limiting, meaning that it will ultimately go away.

Alexander technique – a system of postural awareness.

Bowen technique – a method of holistic massage, as originated by the late Tom Bowen.

Cervical – the neck area.

Chiropractor – a practitioner of a form of manipulative therapy called chiropractic. The title is protected by Act of Parliament.

Chronic pain – persistent pain that is not going to go away of its own accord.

Disc – a structure rather like a car tyre that separates two vertebrae of the spinal column and acts like a shock absorber.

Dorn Method – a gentle manual therapy which is gradually gaining popularity in the UK.

Endorphin – a natural painkilling chemical manufactured by the body.

Homoeopathy – a therapeutic system of medicine using preparations of substances whose effects when administered to healthy subjects correspond to the manifestations of the disorder in the individual patient. The method was developed by Samuel Hahnemann (1755 to 1843) and is now practised throughout the world.

The human pain matrix – a widespread neurological network throughout the central nervous system and brain that is involved in the perception of all types of pain.

Kyphosis – a backward curve of the spine. If this is excessive in the thoracic or chest area of the spine it can produce a humpback appearance.

The Life Cycle – a concept that allows the individual to look at the different aspects of their life, including physical symptoms, emotions, thoughts, behaviour, lifestyle and relationships, in an organised manner, in order to see how modification of different aspects can offer multiple strategies for dealing with any chronic problem.

Ligament – a small tough band of tissue that connects the ends of bones together to form joints. They have a supporting and buffering function and also limit the movements of joints.

Lordosis – the forward curve of the lower back.

Lumbago – a non-specific name for low back pain.

Lumbar – the lower back between the pelvis and the chest.

Neuromuscular system – the muscles of the whole locomotor system and their nerve supplies.

Orthopaedic medicine – a speciality of medicine, which diagnoses and treats non-surgical conditions of the musculoskeletal system with a variety of manipulative techniques; dry needling or acupuncture, joint injections, injection of local anaesthetic or steroids, and other high-tech treatments.

Osteomyologist – a practitioner of massage and manipulative therapy; a qualified member of the Association of Osteomyology.

Osteopath – a practitioner of a manipulative form of therapy. The title is protected by Act of Parliament.

Physiotherapist – a qualified practitioner of physiotherapy. Physiotherapists use a variety of physical treatments to help people with a whole range of physical conditions. They use massage and manipulation with their hands to relieve muscle pains and stiffness and to help the circulation to various parts of the body. They also use heat, cold, electrical current, ultrasound, light treatment and hydrotherapy. Very importantly, they are experts in the use of remedial exercise, which is generally tailored to the individual's needs.

Prolapse – this is a process in which a body part has slipped out of position. In the context of a prolapsed intervertebral disc, the inner jelly-like material seeps through the fibrous ring to cause pressure on nearby nerves.

Psychoneuroimmunology (PNI) – the term refers to the interaction of the mind (psyche), the nervous system (neuro) and the immune system. It demonstrates how stress can affect other systems of the body.

Recurrent pain – this is the name given to acute pain in repeated episodes. This is the type that you get with repeated attacks of back pain.

Rheumatoid arthritis – a very specific type of inflammatory arthritis. It is characterised by specific changes in the blood. It usually requires specialised medical treatment.

Rolfing – also known as Structural Integration, this is a form of bodywork that reorganises the connective tissues, called fascia, that permeate the entire body.

Rubefacient – a rubbing agent, e.g. an ointment, liniment or embrocation which produces a warming effect on the skin to help relieve deeper pain.

Sciatica – pain radiating from the back down the leg, as a result of pressure on nerve roots of the sciatic nerve.

Scoliosis – a sidewards curve of the spine, which may also result in a twist that pulls the ribcage out of position.

Thoracic – the area of the spine that forms the chest.

Three curves – a healthy back has three natural curves: a slight forward curve in the neck (cervical curve), a slight backward curve in the upper back (thoracic curve), and a slight forward curve in the low back (lumbar curve).

Trunk – the name given to the torso, or to the chest and the abdomen.

Vertebrae – the individual bones of the spinal column.

Helpful Reading

Darlington, Gail and Gamlin, Linda, *Diet and Arthritis: A Comprehensive Guide to Controlling Arthritis Through Diet* (BCA, 1998). An excellent and thorough examination of the benefit of diet and dietary change on arthritis, which may also be helpful to people with chronic back pain.

Egoscue, Pete, *Pain Free: A Revolutionary Method for Stopping Chronic Pain* (Bantam Books, 1998). This book looks at exercises that can be done to reduce and prevent pain. It is particularly good on back pain.

Hills, Margaret, *Curing Arthritis the Drug-free Way* (Sheldon Press, 1985). This book has been a best-seller for many years. It looks at the use of cider vinegar, honey and Epsom salt baths to treat arthritis.

Key, Sarah, *Sarah Key's Back Sufferers' Bible* (Vermillion, 2000). A useful book to help understand the way the spine works with methods of helping yourself.

Kingsley, Noel, *Perfect Poise, Perfect Life* (Hodder, 2005). An excellent book that uses the Alexander technique to help you balance your posture and achieve better overall balance in your life.

Melzack, Ronald and Wall, Patrick D, *The Challenge of Pain*, (2nd edition, Penguin Books, 2008). For anyone wanting to understand the nature of chronic pain. A classic book by two of the most outstanding pain scientists in the world.

Romaine, Deborah S and DeWitt, Dawn E, *The Complete Idiot's Guide to Healing Back Pain* (Alpha Books, 1999). A good overview of all the things that can cause back pain and the different treatments available.

Souter, Keith, *Homoeopathy for the Third Age: Treatment for People In Middle and Later Life* (CW Daniels Co, 1993). A general text on homoeopathic treatments for a range of conditions.

Wilson, Andrew, *The Complete Guide to Good Posture at Work* (Vermillion, 1996). An excellent book covering posture and the problems that can result from faulty posture, specifically as it relates to the work environment.

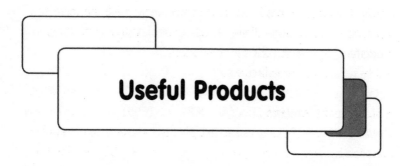

Useful Products

Below is a list of products and suppliers of products that may help to ease back pain. The author does not endorse or recommend any particular product and this list is by no means exhaustive.

Aloe Vera
Either taken as juice or as a capsule in a dose of 200 mg per day seems to be helpful in reducing pain, inflammation and stiffness.
Website: www.aloe-vera2u.co.uk

Biofreeze Pain Relieving Gel
Herbal preparations to rub on which may help to soothe aching back muscles.
Website: www.biofreeze.co.uk

Boots St John's Wort
Hypericum (the Latin name for St John's Wort) can be an effective mild anti-depressant. You should tell your doctor you are taking it, especially if you are taking the oral contraceptive pill or any prescribed drugs.
Website: www.boots.com

Boswellia serrata

Indian frankincense has been used in Ayurvedic medicine for many centuries. It has anti-inflammatory properties that may help if underlying arthritis is causing the back pain.

Website: www.ayurvediccure.com

Calcium and Vitamin D

A daily dose of this reduces the risk of osteoporosis. It is obtainable over the counter from any pharmacist and can also be prescribed by your doctor.

Copper Bracelets

There seems to be some evidence that these may help some people with back pain. They can also contain magnets.

Website: www.magnets4health.co.uk

Deep Heat

A traditional embrocation, containing mentholatum to produce a warming effect on painful muscles.

Website: www.mentholatum.co.uk

Epsom Salts

An Epsom salt bath is often useful in easing an aching back. Must not be taken internally.

Website: www.justasoap.co.uk

Essential oils

Arnica, sage, cedarwood, lavender, camomile or juniper oils may be added to a bath and may be helpful.

Website: www.justaromatherapy.co.uk

Ginger

Powdered ginger can be taken in food or as a supplement.
Website: www.nutricentre.com

Glucosamine and Chondroitin Complex

This may be helpful if the underlying cause of back pain is arthritis.
Do not take this if allergic to seafood, or if taking anti-coagulants.
Website: www.nutricentre.com

Inversion tables

These work on the principle that if you are inverted or suspended
upside down then gravity will produce a traction effect to decompress
the spine.
Website: www.inversiontableuk.com

Magnets

There are various types of magnets that many people find useful.
Magnetic bracelets, or special body wraps with magnets inside them
are available. Also copper bracelets with magnets inside them are
available.
Website: www.magnets4health.co.uk

MSM

Methylsulfonylmethane is a useful supplement of sulphur and is
anti-inflammatory. Avoid if allergic to sulphur or sulphates.
Website: www.nutricentre.com

Quercetin

This is an effective anti-oxidant found in apples, onions and tea. A
daily supplement of 500mg daily may be generally beneficial and
may reduce inflammation.
Website: www.naturesbest.co.uk

SBC Arnica – gel

Arnica gel is a useful embrocation.
Website: www.salonskincare.co.uk

SBC Intensive Arnica Warming gel

This gel contains arnica and has a pleasant warming effect. It must be washed off afterwards and could stain clothing.
Website: www.salonskincare.co.uk

Sore No More

Natural herbal preparations including aloe vera, capsaicin, camphor, green tea and witch hazel, which can be applied to the back and may help aching pains.
Website: www.sorenomore.com

Twinings Nettle and Fennel Tea

Many people with chronic back pain find nettle tea helpful. A cup twice a day.
Website: www.twinings.co.uk

Vegetarian Glucosamine

This is glucosamine derived from corn. It is suitable for vegetarians and anyone allergic to seafood.
Website: www.naturesbest.co.uk

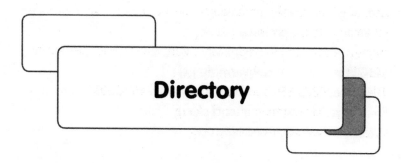

Directory

Alliance of Registered Homeopaths

The ARH is a professional organisation that supports and promotes a high standard of safe, effective homeopathic practices. A free copy of the ARH Register of qualified homeopaths can be obtained using the contact details below.

Address: Millbrook, Millbrook Hill, Nutley, East Sussex, TN22 3PJ
Telephone: 01825 714506
Email: info@a-r-h.org
Website: www.a-r-h.org

Arthritis Care

Arthritis Care supports people with arthritis. It is the UK's largest organisation working with and for all people who have arthritis.

Address: 18 Stephenson Way, London, NW1 2HD
Helpline: 0808 800 4050
Telephone: 020 7380 6500
Email: info@arthritiscare.org.uk
Website: www.arthritiscare.org.uk

Arthritis Research UK

The Arthritis Research Campaign (ARC), founded in 1936, raises funds to promote medical research into the cause, treatment and cure of arthritic conditions; to educate medical students, doctors and allied healthcare professionals about arthritis; and provide information to the general public.

Address: Copeman House St Mary's Gate, Chesterfield, Derbyshire, S41 7TD

Telephone: 0870 850 5000 (UK only) or 01246 558033

Email: enquiries@arthritisresearchuk.org

Website: www.arthritisresearchuk.org

The Association of Osteomyologists

The Association of Osteomyologists represents practitioners of several related therapies, which treat nerve, bone and muscle problems, using a range of manipulative and massage techniques, often coupled with advice on nutrition and daily living. Practitioners are educated to degree and postgraduate level and are usually members of the Association of Osteomyology.

Address: 80 Greenstead Avenue, Woodford Green, Essex, IG8 7ER

Telephone: 0208 504 1462

Email: info@osteomyology.co.uk

Website: www.osteomyology.co.uk

BackCare

BackCare is a national charity that aims to reduce the impact of back pain on society by providing information, support, promoting good practice and funding research. BackCare acts as a hub between patients, (healthcare) professionals, employers, policy makers, researchers and all others with an interest in back pain.

Address: 16 Elmtree Road, Teddington, TW11 8ST

Helpline: 0845 130 2704

Telephone (main office): 0208 977 5474

Website: www.backcare.org.uk

Benefit Enquiry Line

Benefit Enquiry Line provides advice and information for disabled people and carers on the range of benefits available.

Address: 2nd Floor, Red Rose House, Lancaster Road, Preston, Lancashire, PR1 1HB

Telephone: 0900 882 200

Textphone: 0800 243 355

Email: BEL-Customer-Services@dwp.gsi.gov.uk

Website: www.direct.gov.uk/disability-money

The British Acupuncture Council

The British Acupuncture Council (BAcC) is the leading self-regulatory body for the practise of traditional acupuncture in the UK

Address: 63 Jeddo Road, London, W12 9HQ

Telephone: 020 8735 0400

Fax: 020 8735 0404

Website: www.acupuncture.org.uk

The British Chiropractic Association (BCA)

The BCA is the largest and longest-established association for chiropractors in the UK. It represents over 50 per cent of UK chiropractors. All BCA chiropractors will have undergone an internationally-accredited undergraduate course and are registered with the General Chiropractic Council, the UK's statutory regulator for the profession. The BCA aim to promote, encourage and maintain high standards of conduct, practice, education and training within the profession in the UK.

Address: 59 Castle Street, Reading, Berkshire, RG1 7SN

Telephone: 0118 950 5950

Fax: 0118 958 8946

Email: enquiries@chiropractic-uk.co.uk

Website: www.chiropractic-uk.co.uk

The British Medical Acupuncture Society (BMAS)

The British Medical Acupuncture Society is a registered charity established to encourage the use and scientific understanding of acupuncture within medicine for the public benefit. It seeks to enhance the education and training of suitably qualified practitioners, and to promote high standards of working practices in acupuncture. Members are regulated healthcare professionals who practise acupuncture within the scope of their professional practice.

The BMAS has two offices, one based in Northwich and one in London:

Northwich Office:

Address: BMAS House, 3 Winnington Court, Northwich, Cheshire, CW8 1AQ

Telephone: 01606 786782

London Office:

Address: BMAS, Royal London Homoeopathic Hospital, 60 Great Ormond Street, London, WC1N 3HR

Telephone: 020 7713 9437

Email: bmaslondon@aol.com

Website: www.medical-acupuncture.co.uk

The British Wheel of Yoga (BWY)

The British Wheel of Yoga is a registered charity and is the largest yoga organisation in the country, running for 40 years. It is the Governing Body, and accredits other yoga teacher training organisations.

Address: BWY Central Office, British Wheel of Yoga, 25 Jermyn Street, Sleaford, Lincolnshire, NG34 7RU

Telephone: 01529 306851

Fax: 01529 303233

Email: office@bwy.org.uk

Website: www.bwy.org.uk

The Chartered Society of Physiotherapy (CSP)

The Chartered Society of Physiotherapy is the professional, educational and trade union body for the UK's 49,000 chartered physiotherapists, physiotherapy students and assistants.
Address: 14 Bedford Row, London, WC1R 4ED
Telephone: 020 7306 6666
Website: www.csp.org.uk

Disabled Living Foundation

DLF is a national charity that provides impartial advice, information and training on daily living aids.
Address: 380–384 Harrow Road, London, W9 2HU
Helpline: 0845 130 9177 (textphone: 020 7432 8009)
Telephone (switchboard): 020 7289 6111
Email: helpline@dlf.org.uk or info@dlf.org.uk
Website: www.dlf.org.uk

Faculty of Homeopathy

The Faculty of Homeopathy promotes the academic and scientific development of homeopathy and ensures the highest standards in the education, training and practice of homeopathy by statutorily registered healthcare professionals. This includes doctors, dentists, nurses, veterinary surgeons, midwives, pharmacists and podiatrists, all of whom have taken further training in homeopathy.
Address: Hahnemann House, 29 Park Street West, Luton, LU1 3BE
Telephone: 01582 408680
Fax: 01582 723032
Website: www.facultyofhomeopathy.org

Fibromyalgia Association UK

Fibromyalgia Association UK is a registered charity which was established in order to provide information and support to sufferers

and their families. In addition, the Association provides medical information for professionals and operates a national helpline.
Address: PO Box 206, Stourbridge, West Midlands, DY9 8YL
Helpline: 0845 345 2322
Benefit helpline: 0845 345 2343
Telephone: 01384 895 002
Email: charity@fmauk.org
Website: www.fibromyalgia-associationuk.org

General Osteopathic Council
The General Osteopathic Council regulates the practice of osteopathy in the United Kingdom. By law osteopaths must be registered with the GOC in order to practise in the UK.
Address:176 Tower Bridge Road, London, SE1 3LU
Telephone: 020 7357 6655
Fax: 020 7357 0011
Email: contactus@osteopathy.org.uk
Website: www.osteopathy.org.uk

The Institute of Sport and Remedial Massage (ISRM)
The Institute of Sport and Remedial Massage aims to unite independent schools of sport and remedial massage under a single, externally validated Sport & Remedial Massage qualification, ensuring quality of training. The ISRM represents therapists who employ a range of assessment and remedial techniques to effectively treat a variety of soft tissue conditions.
Address: 28 Station Parade, Willesden Green, London, NW2 4NX
Telephone: 020 8450 5851
Email: admin@theisrm.com
Website: www.theisrm.com

The National Institute of Medical Herbalists (NIMH)

The National Institute of Medical Herbalists is the UK's leading professional body representing herbal practitioners. The Institute maintains a register of individual members, sets the profession's educational standards and runs an accreditation system for training establishments.

Address: Elm House, 54 Mary Arches Street, Exeter, EX4 3BA

Telephone: 01392 426 022

Fax: 01392 498 963

Email: info@nimh.org.uk

Website: www.nimh.org.uk

NHS Wheelchair Service

It is possible to get a wheelchair through the NHS Wheelchair Service. These services are run by local health authorities so the services provided and organisation varies.

The Wheelchair Service provides appropriate mobility equipment for people of all ages with a long-term disability who have difficulty walking and there is usually provision for short-term loan wheelchairs. An assessment is included to ensure needs are met.

NHS Directory of wheelchair services: www.wheelchairmanagers. nhs.uk/services.asp

Website:

www.direct.gov.uk/en/DisabledPeople/HealthAndSupport

The Reflexology Forum

The Reflexology Forum is the developing regulatory body in the UK for reflexology. It is a means whereby organisations with reflexologists on their register can have a voice as to how reflexology develops in this country. There are several organisations within reflexology which are affiliated with it, including the Association of Reflexologists, British

Reflexology Association, the Clinical Association of Reflexologists and the International Federation of Reflexologists.
Address: Dalton House, 60 Windsor Avenue, London, SW19 2RR
Telephone: 0800 037 0130
Email: pr@reflexologyforum.org
Website: www.reflexologyforum.org

The Scoliosis Association (UK) (SAUK)

SAUK aims to provide advice, support and information to people with scoliosis and to raise awareness among health professionals and the general public.
Address: 4 Ivebury Court, 323–327 Latimer Road, London, W10 6RA
Helpline: 020 8964 1166
Telephone: 020 8964 5343
Email: sauk@sauk.org.uk
Website: www.scoliosis.org.uk

The Society of Homeopaths

The Society of Homeopaths is the largest organisation registering professional homeopaths in Europe.
Address:11 Brookfield, Duncan Close, Moulton Park, Northampton, NN3 6WL
Telephone: 0845 450 6611
Email: info@homeopathy-soh.org
Website: www.homeopathy-soh.org

Society of Orthopaedic Medicine (SOM)

Orthopaedic medicine is the examination, diagnosis and treatment of non-surgical lesions of the musculoskeletal system. The Society of Orthopaedic Medicine was formed in 1979 to develop the work of Dr James Cyriax and to promote the theory and practice of orthopaedic medicine. Membership consists of approximately 1700 doctors and physiotherapists.

Address: 4th Floor, 151 Dale Street, Liverpool, L2 2AH

Telephone: 0151 237 3970

Website: www.somed.org

The Society of Teachers of the Alexander Technique (STAT)

The Alexander technique has been taught for over one hundred years. In 1958, STAT was founded in the UK by teachers who were trained personally by F. M. Alexander. STAT's first aim is to ensure the highest standards of teacher training and professional practice.

Address: 1st Floor, Linton House, 39–51 Highgate Road, London NW5 1RS

Telephone: 0207 482 5135

Email: office@stat.org.uk

Website: www.stat.org.uk

The T'ai Chi Union for Great Britain

The T'ai Chi Union for Great Britain is an association of practitioners of recognised styles of T'ai Chi Chuan. It was founded in 1991 and has grown to include a national list of over 800 registered instructors throughout the whole of the British Isles.

It exists to unite T'ai Chi practitioners, promote T'ai Chi in all its aspects including health, aesthetic meditation and self-defence.

Address (Secretary): Peter Ballam, 5 Corunna Drive, Horsham, West Sussex, RH13 5HG

Telephone (Secretary): 01403 257 918

Email (Secretary): PeterBallam@aol.com

Address (Membership): 18 Branziert Road, North Killeam, Stirlingshire, G63 9RF

Telephone (Membership): 01360 550 461

Email (Membership): bumper@lineone.net

Website: www.taichiunion.com